Pediatric Traumatic Emergencies

What Do I Do Now?: Emergency Medicine

SERIES EDITORS-IN-CHIEF

Catherine A. Marco, MD, FACEP
Professor, Emergency Medicine & Surgery
Wright State University Boonshoft School of Medicine
Dayton, Ohio

OTHER VOLUMES IN THE SERIES
Pediatric Medical Emergencies

FORTHCOMING VOLUMES
Legal and Ethical Issues in Emergency Medicine
Critical Care Emergencies

Pediatric Traumatic Emergencies

Edited by
Ann M. Dietrich, MD, FAAP, FACEP
Associate Professor of Pediatrics
Ohio University
Heritage College of Medicine
Medical Director of Education
Ohio ACEP
Columbus, OH

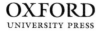

OXFORD
UNIVERSITY PRESS

OXFORD
UNIVERSITY PRESS

Oxford University Press is a department of the University of Oxford. It furthers
the University's objective of excellence in research, scholarship, and education
by publishing worldwide. Oxford is a registered trade mark of Oxford University
Press in the UK and certain other countries.

Published in the United States of America by Oxford University Press
198 Madison Avenue, New York, NY 10016, United States of America.

Library of Congress Cataloging-in-Publication Data
Names: Dietrich, Ann M., author.
Title: Pediatric traumatic emergencies / Ann M. Dietrich.
Description: New York, NY : Oxford University Press, [2020] |
Includes bibliographical references and index.
Identifiers: LCCN 2019059640 (print) | LCCN 2019059641 (ebook) |
ISBN 9780190946623 (paperback) | ISBN 9780190946647 (epub) |
ISBN 9780190946654
Subjects: LCSH: Pediatric emergencies. | Children—Wounds and injuries—Treatment.
Classification: LCC RJ370 .D54 2020 (print) | LCC RJ370 (ebook) |
DDC 618.92/0025—dc23
LC record available at https://lccn.loc.gov/2019059640
LC ebook record available at https://lccn.loc.gov/2019059641

9 8 7 6 5 4 3 2 1
Printed by Marquis, Canada

Contents

Contributors

Isabel A. Barata, MS, MD, MBA, FACP, FAAP, FACEP
Professor of Pediatrics and
Emergency Medicine
Donald and Barbara Zucker
School of Medicine at Hofstra/
Northwell
Pediatric Emergency Medicine
Service Line Quality Director
Emergency Medicine and Pediatrics
Service Line
Director of Pediatric Emergency
Medicine
North Shore University Hospital
Manhasset, NY

Elizabeth A. Berdan, MD, MS
Pediatric Surgery
Mary Bridge Children's Hospital &
Health Network
President, American Medical
Women's Association—
Physicians Against the
Trafficking of Humans
(AMWA-PATH)

Kristol Das, MD
Assistant Professor
Department of Emergency
Medicine
Nationwide Children's Hospital
Columbus, OH

Carrie DeHoff, MD
Department of Emergency
Medicine
Nationwide Children's Hospital
Ohio State University
Columbus, OH

Woo Do, MD
Resident, Department of Surgery
Madigan Army Medical Center
Tacoma, WA

Evan Feinberg, MD
Department of Emergency
Medicine
Northwell Health at Long Island
Jewish Medical Center and
North Shore University
Hospital
New Hyde Park, NY, and
Manhasset, NY

Christie Gutierrez, MD
Pediatric Emergency
Medicine Fellow
Columbia University
Medical Center
New York, NY

Shilpa Hari, MD
Department of Pediatrics
Staten Island University Hospital
Staten Island, NY

John Horton, MD
Department of Surgery
Madigan Army Medical Center
Tacoma, WA
Assistant Professor
Department of Surgery
Uniformed Services University
Bethesda, MD

Angela Hua, MD
Assistant Professor
Department of Emergency
  Medicine
Donald and Barbara Zucker
  School of Medicine at
  Hofstra/Northwell
Emergency Medicine Department
  Faculty
Long Island Jewish
  Medical Center
New Hyde Park, NY

Victor Huang, MD
Primary Care Sports Medicine
  Fellow
Department of Emergency
  Medicine
North Shore University Hospital
Northwell Health System
Manhasset, NY

Julianne Hughes, MD
Pediatric Emergency
  Medicine Fellow
Nemours/Alfred I. duPont Hospital
  for Children
Wilmington, DE

Kaileen Jafari
Pediatric Emergency
  Medicine Fellow
Seattle Children's Hospital/
  University of Washington
  Medical Center
Seattle, WA

Nima Jalali, MD
Primary Care Sports Medicine
  Fellow
Department of Emergency Medicine
North Shore University Hospital
Manhasset, NY

Dana Kaplan, MD
Director of Child Abuse and
  Neglect
Medical Director
Staten Island CAC
Associate Program Director
  Pediatrics Residency Training
  Program
Department of Pediatrics
Staten Island University Hospital
Assistant Professor of Pediatrics
Donald and Barbara Zucker
  School of Medicine at Hofstra
  Northwell
Staten Island, NY

Anisha Khaitan, MD
Pediatric Emergency
  Medicine Fellow
Columbia University
  Medical Center
New York, NY

Danny Lammers, MD
Resident, Department of Surgery
Madigan Army Medical Center
Tacoma, WA

Seth Linakis, MD, MA
Division of Pediatric Emergency
    Medicine
Nationwide Children's Hospital
Columbus, OH

Laurie Malia, DO
Assistant Professor of Pediatrics in
    Emergency Medicine
Columbia University Medical
    Center, Morgan Stanley
    Children's Hospital
New York, NY

Christopher Marenco, MD
General Surgery Resident,
    Department of Surgery
Madigan Army Medical Center
Tacoma, WA

**Bryan McCarty, MD,
CAQSM, FACEP**
Department of Emergency
    Medicine
Northwell Health System
North Shore University Hospital
Manhasset, NY

Melissa A. McGuire, MD
Assistant Professor
Department of Emergency Medicine
Northwell Health at North Shore
    University Hospital and Cohen
    Children's Medical Center
Zucker School of Medicine at
    Hofstra/Northwell
Manhasset, NY

Jennifer E. Melvin, MD
Assistant Professor of Pediatrics
Department of Emergency Medicine
Nationwide Children's Hospital
Columbus, OH

Ajay K. Puri, MD
Resident
Department of Emergency Medicine
Northwell Health at North Shore
    University Hospital and Long
    Island Jewish Medical Center
Manhasset, NY

Joni E. Rabiner, MD
Associate Professor of Pediatrics in
    Emergency Medicine
Columbia University Medical
    Center, Morgan Stanley
    Children's Hospital
New York, NY

Mir Raza, MD, PGY3
Department of Emergency Medicine
Northwell Health at North Shore
    University Hospital and Long
    Island Jewish Medical Center
Manhasset, NY

Lara Reda, MD
Assistant Professor of Emergency
    Medicine
Donald and Barbara Zucker
    School of Medicine at Hofstra/
    Northwell
Manhasset, NY

Nancy Rixe, MD
Pediatric Emergency
    Medicine Fellow
UPMC Children's Hospital of
    Pittsburgh
Pittsburgh, PA

Hoi See Tsao, MD, FAAP
Pediatric Emergency
    Medicine Fellow
Hasbro Children's Hospital
The Alpert Medical School of
    Brown University
Providence, RI

**Philipp J. Underwood, MD,
FAAEM, FACEP, FAAFP**
Program Director
Sports Medicine Fellowship
Department of Emergency
    Medicine
North Shore University Hospital
Manhasset, NY

**Jessica J. Wall, MD, MPH,
MSCE, NREMT-P**
Clinical Assistant Professor of
    Emergency Medicine and Pediatrics
University of Washington, School
    of Medicine
Associate Pediatric Medical
    Director, Airlift Northwest
Seattle Children's Hospital, Division
    of Pediatric Emergency Medicine
Harborview Medical Center,
    Department of Emergency Medicine
Seattle, WA

Robyn Wing, MD, MPH, FAAP
Assistant Professor of Emergency
    Medicine and Pediatrics
Hasbro Children's Hospital, The
    Alpert Medical School of Brown
    University
Providence, RI

Walter Wiswell, MD
Emergency Medicine Resident
Department of Emergency Medicine
North Shore University Hospital
Northwell Health System
Manhasset, NY

Elizabeth A. Woods, MD
Medical Director
Child Abuse Intervention Department
Mary Bridge Children's Hospital &
    Health Network
Clinical Assistant Professor
Department of Pediatrics
Uniformed Services University of
    Health Sciences
Bethesda, MD

1 Too Much Contact

Christie Gutierrez and Anisha Khaitan

An 8-year-old girl is found lying on the grass after being struck by a moving vehicle on a busy main street. An adult bystander tells you that she saw the patient hit from the front by a moving vehicle from her living room window. Nobody has moved her.

Initial assessment shows that the girl is responding only to painful stimuli. Breathing is shallow with audible snoring. The skin is pale with mild cyanosis. Respiratory rate is 10 breaths per minute. Heart rate is 140 beats per minute. The skin is cold, radial pulses are thready, and capillary refill is >3 seconds. Pupils are equally dilated and are reactive to light. Poor air entry is auscultated on the left, and diminished air entry is heard on the right. Oxygen saturation is 82%.

She has multiple broken teeth and is bleeding from her upper lip. The abdomen is stiff on palpation. She has extensive bruising on her torso. The left leg is swollen with evident deformity to the left femur.

What do you do now?

DISCUSSION

General Considerations

Trauma is the number one cause of death in children ages 1 through 18 years in the United States. It accounts for greater than 50% of childhood deaths. The most common traumatic injuries in children are head injuries, thoracic injuries, abdominal trauma, and extremity injuries. Head trauma is the leading cause of death in pediatric multitrauma patients.

Management of the pediatric trauma patient requires a systematic approach for initial evaluation, stabilization, and treatment. The primary survey, modified for the pediatric patient, is designed to provide healthcare providers with a systematic and protocolized approach to managing trauma patients. The primary survey is followed by the secondary survey to complete a head-to-toe examination of the patient.

PRIMARY SURVEY

The goal of the primary survey is to perform an initial evaluation of the patient to quickly identify and treat life-threatening conditions. The 5 parts of the primary survey constitute the ABCDE approach: Airway Maintenance, Breathing and Ventilation, Circulation, Disability (i.e., neurologic status), and Exposure/Environment.

Airway—The most important first step in the management of pediatric trauma patients is the assessment and stabilization of the airway. The goal is to recognize and to correct obstruction, to prevent gastric content aspiration, and to optimize gas exchange. Remember that children desaturate more quickly than adults, which can lead to respiratory arrest, and then to cardiac arrest. Start by assessing the patency of the airway, making note of whether the child has increased work of breathing, poor chest rise, or completely absent respirations. Is there evidence of a hoarse cry, stridor, or muted voice?

Determine whether the airway is stable and provide airway maneuvers as needed, such as jaw thrust, nasal or oral suctioning, or use of airway adjuncts like nasal trumpets, oral airways, or supraglottic devices. If unable to maintain the airway with these maneuvers, consider endotracheal tube placement with rapid sequence intubation. It is important to remember when managing the airway that trauma patients can have cervical spine injuries, so maintain in-line cervical spine stabilization with a hard cervical collar.

Some airway-related anatomic and physiologic characteristics specific to children are:

- A prominent occiput may lead to neck flexion on a flat surface during airway management.
- The larger tongue to mandible ratio can make bag mask ventilation and intubation more difficult in children.
- Younger children have a more flexible anterior-placed, omega-shaped epiglottis, which may require a straight blade to lift epiglottis (e.g., Miller blade) to visualize the vocal cords.
- Younger patients have higher respiratory rates and increased amounts of secretions.
- Infants less than 3 months of age are obligate nasal breathers, which makes them more vulnerable to anatomic obstructions and infection.

Special considerations when evaluating the airway include special attention to patients with facial or neck trauma, facial burns, or neurologic injury that compromise a patient's ability to protect their airway. Indications for endotracheal intubation in a trauma patient include:

- Glasgow coma score <8 or inability to maintain or protect the airway
- Inadequate oxygenation or ventilation
- Inability to ventilate or oxygenate with bag valve mask
- Potential for clinical deterioration (e.g., facial burns, inhalation injury)
- Decompensated shock resistant to fluid resuscitation
- Anticipated surgical intervention or need for radiologic investigation outside of the ED in an unstable patient

Based on the patient scenario the child has audible snoring and cyanosis. Immediate inline stabilization of the spine should be achieved with a jaw thrust to attempt to open the airway. With the cyanosis and poor chest movement immediate initiation of bag-valve-mask ventilation would be appropriate with 100% oxygen.

Breathing—After the airway assessment is complete, the next step is to evaluate for breathing, which is the preservation of oxygenation and ventilation. To evaluate the patient's breathing, inspect, auscultate, and palpate. Look for thoracic movements (rate, depth, and pattern of breathing), tracheal deviation, work of breathing, symmetry of chest wall movement (e.g., assessing for flail chest, pneumothorax, or hemothorax), and skin color. When auscultating, assess for signs of upper airway obstruction (e.g., stridor), signs of pneumothorax/hemothorax, and air movement. It is important to remember that younger children are predominantly diaphragmatic breathers, so they are more sensitive to intra-abdominal pressures than older children or adults.

Some anatomic characteristics specific to children with effects on breathing are:

- Increased transmission of blunt forces to the lung parenchyma secondary to the high compliance of the pediatric rib cage leads to an increased incidence of pulmonary contusions, pneumothorax, and hemothorax in this population and a lower incidence of rib fractures.
- The diameter of pediatric airways is smaller than that of adults, so any change in the lumen diameter secondary to fluids, secretions, or inflammation can significantly increase the risk of airway obstruction. These structures are also more vulnerable to barotrauma from excessive volume ventilation during resuscitation.

This child is receiving bag-valve-mask (BVM) ventilation. There are no bruises or evidence of trauma to the child's chest. Breath sounds are much improved with BVM and equal bilaterally. Skin color has also improved.

Circulation—In a pediatric polytrauma patient, it is critical to recognize early signs of shock. These signs include tachycardia for age, followed by delayed capillary refill, skin mottling, cool extremities, and altered mental status. In children, cardiac output is reflective of heart rate, so significant blood loss is associated with profound tachycardia. Pediatric patients will not initially become hypotensive, as they are generally able to adjust vascular tone to preferentially perfuse core organs. Hypotension is a late vital sign change, occurring only after 25%–30% of circulating blood volume is lost, and is often indicative of significant cardiovascular compromise and decompensated shock. Decompensated shock can quickly lead to cardiopulmonary failure. Pediatric Advanced Life Support (PALS) recommends early fluid resuscitation with crystalloid and blood products as needed for trauma patients.

Some circulation-related physiologic characteristics specific to children are:

- Pediatric patients have less fluid reserve, which predisposes them to dehydration.
- Children have less circulating blood volume, so small amounts of blood loss can lead to hypovolemic shock.
- Fluid resuscitation with isotonic solution is based on weight. For shock, give rapid crystalloid fluid boluses of 20 mL/kg. If three boluses of crystalloid is insufficient, consider giving aliquots of 10 mL/kg of blood (O-negative pRBCs) if the child is persistently hypotensive after initial crystalloid fluid resuscitation.
- The child in the case shows clear signs of circulatory compromise, tachycardia, cold skin, thready peripheral pulses, and a capillary refill greater than 3 seconds.

Disability—Disability is a quick neurologic assessment of a patient to determine the state of consciousness, mental status, and neurologic deficits. This evaluation includes mental status evaluation using the modified pediatric Glasgow Coma Scale (level of alertness, response to verbal or painful stimuli, pupillary response) and motor exam (to determine whether the patient has motor activity in all four extremities). See Table 1.1 for more details on the pediatric Glasgow coma scale point assignment. To assess the neurologic status while doing a quick gross motor and sensory exam, PALS also recommends using the AVPU mnemonic: Alert—fully alert, Voice—responds to voice, Pain—responds to pain, and Unresponsive—is completely unresponsive.

The goal is to identify early signs of head injury and address any hypoxia or perfusion deficits to prevent the development of secondary cerebral injury or increased intracranial pressures (ICP). General recommendations

TABLE 1.1. **Pediatric Glasgow Coma Scale**

	Glasgow Coma Scale	**Infant Coma Scale**	**Score**
Eye Opening	Spontaneous	Spontaneous	4
	To voice	To voice	3
	To pain	To pain	2
	None	None	1
Verbal Response	Oriented	Coos, Babbles	5
	Confused	Irritable cry, Consolable	4
	Inappropriate	Cries to pain	3
	Garbled	Moans to pain	2
	None	None	1
Motor Response	Obeys commands	Normal movements	6
	Localizes pain	Withdraws to touch	5
	Withdraws to pain	Withdraws to pain	4
	Flexion	Flexion	3
	Extension	Extension	2
	Flaccid	Flaccid	1

Source: Fleischer et al. 2010.

are to prevent hypotension, hypovolemia, hypoxia, hypothermia, and hypoglycemia.

The patient in the scenario is only responsive to pain. As you assist with BVM her level of responsiveness does not improve.

Environment/Exposure—This last step in the primary survey requires both exposing the child to assess for the full range of potential injuries and making adjustments to the environment to maintain euthermia. Pediatric patients are particularly vulnerable to hypothermia, especially infants, who have large surface-area-to-volume ratios. Pay close attention to the body temperature of the patient during the initial assessment and throughout the resuscitation. If the patient becomes hypothermic, consider measures to maintain euthermia by removing wet clothing, using radiant warmers, and/or infusing warmed intravenous fluids, as appropriate.

Adjuncts to the Primary Survey

Access—Establish venous access preferentially by a peripheral percutaneous route. If unsuccessful after two attempts, in a patient who has evidence of circulatory compromise, attempt an intraosseous infusion. It is difficult to establish intravenous access in children with hypovolemia because of circulatory collapse. Intraosseous placement is a reasonable emergency access procedure in these cases.

Preferred pediatric venous access:

- Percutaneous peripheral—antecubital fossa, saphenous vein at ankle
- Intraosseous placement—anteromedial tibia, distal femur
- Percutaneous placement—femoral veins

The child in the scenario is responsive only to pain, has required ventilatory support (BVM), and has clear evidence of a significantly compromised circulatory status, and therefore an immediate decision is made to place an intraosseous line. The line is placed in the right tibia (should not go below the site of the femur fracture on the left side). A 20 mL/kg fluid bolus is administered as a rapid bolus through the intraosseus (IO) route.

SECONDARY SURVEY

The secondary survey is a systematic head-to-toe examination performed after the primary survey is completed and resuscitation has been initiated. The goal is to identify all of the other injuries the patient may have sustained. Of note, the secondary survey should include repetition of the primary survey, as the patient's condition may have changed since the initial evaluation. The secondary survey includes initial history, detailed physical exam including cervical spine evaluation and clearance, monitoring vital signs and urinary output, obtaining ancillary studies (e.g., labs and imaging), and performing time-sensitive procedures (e.g., tetanus immunization, antibiotics, nasogastric tube (NGT) or orogastric tube (OGT) placement to decompress the stomach, and Foley catheter insertion to monitor urinary output closely). Remember that urinary output varies with age (infant–1 y: 2 mL/kg/h; young children: 1.5 mL/kg/h; older children: 1 mL/kg/h; adolescents who have stopped growing: 0.5—1 mL/kg/h).

History—The history can be elicited from the patient and/or EMS or accompanying family or friends. Use the mnemonic AMPLE (A-Allergies, M-Medications, P-Past Medical History/Pregnancy, L-Last Meal, and

E-Events/Environment Leading to the Injury) to remember the key points of a quick and focused history.

Head-to-Toe Examination

Head—Check pupil size and reactivity. Check extraocular movements and look for nystagmus. Perform a fundoscopic exam looking for papilledema and hemorrhages. Examine the ears for hemotympanum or cerebrospinal fluid otorrhea. Check the nose for signs of perforated nasal septum. Palpate the skull assessing for lacerations, hematomas, or bony step-offs suggesting fracture. Look in the mouth for active bleeding and for signs of affected dentition.

Some anatomic characteristics specific to children are:

- Because the pediatric head is proportionately larger in young children, it is susceptible to closed head injury and large amounts of blood loss (e.g., cephalohematomas, subgaleal hematomas, scalp lacerations)
- Skull fractures can occur more easily in pediatric patients because of their thinner skulls.

The child's head shows obvious bruising on the right temporal side with blood coming from her ear. Pupils are equal and reactive to light. Extraocular motion is unable to be assessed. She has multiple broken teeth and is bleeding from her upper lip.

Neck—With cervical collar in place, examine the patient for neck lacerations, ecchymosis, masses, or tracheal deviation. Be careful not to compromise the airway when examining the neck. *Roll the patient while immobilizing the cervical spine.* Inspect the posterior surface of the patient from head to toe for injuries. Palpate over the cervical, thoracic, lumbar, and sacral spine and paraspinous regions looking for tenderness, bruising, crepitus, step-offs, or obvious deformities.

Patient has an altered mental status, but has no external bruising or step-offs.

Chest—Observe the chest rise and fall. Paradoxical chest movement can suggest flail chest or pneumothorax. Look for lacerations, ecchymosis, or flail segments. Auscultate the lungs looking for asymmetric, diminished, or absent breath sounds. Auscultate the heart listening for murmurs or rubs. Palpate for tenderness or crepitus. Treat tension pneumothorax (absent breath sounds and unstable vital signs) with needle decompression and subsequent chest tube. Place chest tube for pneumothorax or hemothorax.

Some anatomic characteristics specific to children are:

- Pediatric patients are at higher risk for intrathoracic injuries because they have higher chest wall compliance, an anterior heart, mobile structures in the mediastinum, and delicate tracheobronchial structures. For these reasons, children are more susceptible to pulmonary contusions from low impact injuries and barotrauma during ventilation.
- Rib fractures are less common in pediatrics because of increased elasticity. When present, rib fractures suggest a severe mechanism of injury. Of note, mortality increases with higher numbers of rib fractures.
- It is important to remember that pulmonary contusions are the most common injury found in patients who sustain blunt chest trauma, but these patients often do not have external signs of injury.

The chest wall shows no evidence of external bruising, with BVM breath sounds equal bilaterally.

Abdomen—Inspect the abdomen for distension, abrasions, lacerations, ecchymosis, and masses. Listen carefully for bowel sounds. Palpate for tenderness (high positive predictive value for intra-abdominal injury) and hepatosplenomegaly.

Some anatomic characteristics specific to children are:

- Children have larger abdomens and weaker abdominal wall muscles compared to adults. These anatomic differences in combination with the larger relative size of their intra-abdominal organs put pediatric patients at higher risk of solid organ injury from blunt abdominal trauma and hollow viscus injury from acceleration-deceleration injuries (e.g., seat belt injuries).

The abdominal exam reveals a rigid abdomen, even after placement of a nasogastric tube.

Pelvis—Inspect and palpate the pelvis for tenderness, deformity, or instability. Look for signs of perineal hematoma. Check for blood at the urethral meatus. Perform a rectal exam to check sphincter tone and look for blood in the stool.

The pelvis is stable and there is no blood at the urethral meatus. Rectal exam is normal.

Extremities—Inspect and palpate the extremities looking for lacerations, hematomas, or obvious bony deformities. Splint any fracture sites. Apply direct pressure to any actively bleeding sites.

Some anatomic characteristics specific to children are:

- Children's bones are more susceptible to bowing and fracture due to incomplete calcification and the presence of multiple active growth centers.

The left leg is swollen with evident deformity to the left femur. There is no active bleeding and the pulse is present but thready (same in all extremities).

CASE CONCLUSION

The child is intubated using rapid sequence intubation (RSI) and a second IV is started peripherally. The child is given a second fluid bolus and the heart rate and perfusion stabilize. The child's head CT shows an intracerebral bleed. The child's abdominal CT shows a Grade 3 splenic injury. The child is in the pediatric intensive care unit for 5 days, hospitalized for a total of 30 days, and able to return to school 3 months after the injury with some cognitive deficits.

Special considerations for pediatric patients:

- Family presence when possible is important in the management of a pediatric trauma patient. Not only does the presence of a family member increase patient cooperation but also it promotes communication between the family and the medical team.

Further Reading

AAP Committee on Pediatric Emergency Medicine, Council on Injury, Violence, and Poison Prevention, Section on Critical Care, Section on Orthopedics, Section on Surgery, Section on Transport Medicine, Pediatric Trauma Society, Society of Trauma Nurses, Pediatric Committee. Management of pediatric trauma. *Pediatrics*. 2016;138(2):e20161569.

Advanced trauma life support (ATLS): The Ninth Edition. *J Trauma Acute Care Surg*. 2013;74(5):1363–1366.

American College of Surgeons: National Trauma Databank 2013 Annual Pediatric Report. 2013. https://www.facs.org/~/media/files/quality%20programs/trauma/ntdb/ntdb%20pediatric%20annual%20report% 202013.ashx. Accessed January 30, 2019.

Avarello JT, Cantor RM. Pediatric major trauma: an approach to evaluation and management. *Emerg Med Clin North Am*. 2007;25(3):803–36.

Calder BW, Vogel AM, Zhang J, et al. Focused assessment with sonography for trauma in children after blunt abdominal trauma: a multi-institutional analysis. *J Trauma Acute Care Surg*. 2017;83(2):218–24.

Fein DM, Fagan M. Overall approach to trauma in the emergency department. *Pediatrics*. 2018;29(10):479–89.

Fleischer GR, Ludwig S, Bachur RG, Gorelick MH, Ruddy RM, Shaw KN. *Textbook of Pediatric Emergency Medicine*. 6th ed. Philadelphia: Lippincott Williams & Wilkins; 2010.

Garcia VF, Gotschall CS, Eichelberger MR, et al. Rib fractures in children: a marker of severe trauma. *J Trauma*. 1990;30:695–700.

Gutiérrez CE. Pediatric trauma. In: JE Tintinalli et al., eds. *Tintinalli's Emergency Medicine: A Comprehensive Study Guide*. 8th ed. New York, NY: McGraw-Hill; 2016. http://accessmedicine.mhmedical.com.ezproxy.cul.columbia.edu/content.aspx?bookid=1658&sectionid=109384732. Accessed February 8, 2019.

Holmes JF, Kelley KM, Wooton-Gorges SL, et al. Guidelines for the acute medical management of severe traumatic brain injury in infants, children, and adolescents--second edition. *JAMA*. 2012;317(22):2290–2296. PMID: 22217782.

Kochanek PM, et al. Guidelines for the acute medical management of severe traumatic brain injury in infants, children and adolescents—2nd edition. *Pediatr Crit Care Med*. 2012;13(Suppl 1): S1–82.

2 What a Pain in the Neck!

Walter Wiswell and Bryan McCarty

An 8-year-old male presents to the Emergency
Room after being a restrained passenger in a motor
vehicle collision (MVC). He is brought in by EMS on a
backboard with a C-collar already applied; he is then
rolled onto a stretcher. He is crying and talking to his
parents who are beside him. He is complaining of
significant neck pain that he reports is both midline
and paraspinal in location. According to EMS and his
family, he has not displayed any obvious neurological
deficits or altered consciousness since the event.
He has abrasions over his forehead and his right
elbow, and a large bruise over his right knee. There
are no obvious abrasions or bony deformities on
cervical exam. Further physical exam is significant
for full sensation and strength in upper and lower
extremities; however, the patient continues to report
midline neck pain with movement, along with pain
over his right knee. He has no other known medical
problems, and takes no medication at home.

What do you do now?

DISCUSSION

In this case of pediatric blunt trauma with cervical neck pain, there are several concerning features that would prompt further evaluation. The child's neck pain is unable to be considered purely muscular in nature, as he consistently reports midline tenderness on exam. The mechanism of injury was also high-risk, in that the collision resulted in a vehicle rollover. He also has evidence of other multiple other trauma sites on his body, including what could possibly be considered a "distracting" injury over his right knee.

The most significant concern and primary issue to address here is the possibility of a cervical spine injury. This can be in the form of damage to the cervical vertebrae, ligaments, or the spinal cord itself. Cervical spine injuries in children are extremely rare, occurring in approximately 1%–2% of cases of blunt trauma.[1] However, these injuries, while few and far between, can have significantly negative outcomes if missed; many require surgical intervention, and even when recognized can result in permanent neurological deficits or even death. The most common causes of such injuries are mechanisms classified as severe force (e.g., rollover/high-speed MVC, pedestrian struck, or fall greater than the child's height), axial loading (such as a diving injury), high-speed acceleration/deceleration injuries, and multisystem trauma.[2] The cervical spine is the most common site for spinal injuries in children; however, anatomic difference as children mature result in distinctions in location depending on age. Over three-quarters of all cervical injuries are axial (occiput to C2) in children less than 8 years of age; however, after the age of 8, subaxial (C3–C7) injuries account for more than 50% of cervical spine disruptions.[3]

Immobilization

As in adult trauma, cervical spine immobilization is a common practice in cases of pediatric trauma when possible cervical injury is suspected. The actual studies are limited in terms of improvement in clinical outcomes with cervical motion restriction; however, the overarching consensus is that an attempt to restrict cervical motion and to maintain the spine in a neutral position can decrease rates of spinal cord injury in pediatric trauma patients.[4] The current recommendation is to perform spinal motion restriction in any instance of obvious head or neck injury, multisystem trauma, or altered mental status.

Cervical "immobilization" or "motion restriction" is obtained almost universally in the field via hard C-collar placement when available. Spinal neutral position (i.e., avoiding flexion or extension of the spine) is anatomically age-dependent; under the age of 8, children require an elevation of approximately 1–2 cm to accommodate the larger head size and avoid neck flexion when immobilized (or conversely, a backboard cutout under the head) due to a prominent occiput that forces cervical flexion.[5] However, children greater than 8 years of age require occipital elevation to maintain a neutral spine position (as do adults).

This child was placed on a rigid backboard by EMS. While once considered a standard of care, the evidence supporting their use is extremely limited, and they may be associated with several adverse side-effects, for example, pain, agitation, and difficulty breathing. Currently, the National Association of EMS Physicians and the American College of Surgeons Committee on Trauma does not recommend their routine use. However, in cases of severe trauma where neck pain is significant or neurologic deficits are present, backboards may still be beneficial when applied for transport for brief periods of time.[6]

In this case, the child is reporting midline neck pain with palpation after a high-speed MVC, making placement of a C-collar appropriate. The use of the rigid backboard, as discussed, is controversial, but given the high-risk mechanism of injury and clinically severe cervical neck pain, is not explicitly contraindicated in this case.

Imaging

Once a full physical exam and primary/secondary survey is performed, the next question is whether the patient requires additional spinal imaging to exclude injury.

When to Image

There is not one universally accepted guideline for pediatric cervical spine imaging, and practitioners may pursue imaging based on a combination of clinical presentation, personal training/experience, and gestalt. The decision to image may be made using one, or a combination, of several different clearance guidelines based on patient age and presentation.

In order to help with this process, the Pediatric Emergency Care Applied Research Network (PECARN) conducted a large, multicenter, case-controlled study of children less than 16 years of age to assess factors associated with cervical spine injuries. They found that "altered mental status, focal neurologic findings, neck pain, torticollis, substantial torso injury, conditions predisposing to cervical spine injury, diving, and high-risk motor vehicle crash" increased the risk of having cervical spine injuries; with 98% sensitivity and 26% specificity if a child has 1 or more of these factors.[7]. Additionally, the National Emergency X-ray Utilization Study (NEXUS) and Canadian clinical decision guidelines may be used to help guide decisions (Figure 2.1). While these criteria have been shown to be highly efficacious in adult populations, their applicability in pediatrics is more questionable due to the limited numbers of pediatric patients included in their study demographics. This is especially true for children under the age of 8, whose immature anatomy results in presentations that may differ from adults.[8,9]

In general, the major criteria for further investigation and prompt cervical spine imaging in cases of pediatric trauma are as follows:

- Neck pain
  - Most significantly bony or midline neck tenderness
- Decreased cervical range of motion
- Torticollis
- Altered mental status
  - Regardless of source (e.g., intoxication vs. injury)
- Any reported neurological finding or deficit (EVEN IF TRANSIENT)
- Large, coexisting (distracting) injuries
  - Especially torso injuries
- Conditions predisposing to cervical spine injuries (Trisomy 21, os odontoideum)
- High-risk mechanisms:
  - Motor vehicle collision (head-on collision, rollover, ejected from vehicle, passenger death, or speed >55 miles/hour)
  - Diving
  - Hanging

Trauma Association of Canada (TAC) National Pediatric C-Spine Evaluation Pathway: Reliable[1] Clinical Exam

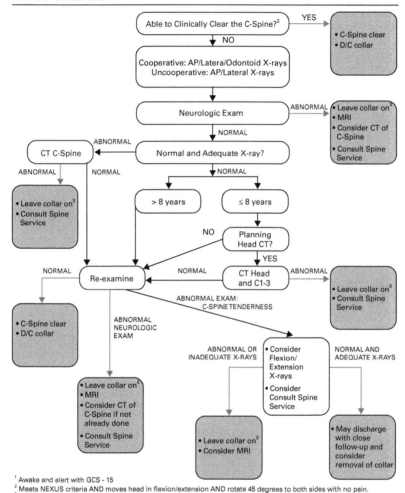

Able to Clinically Clear the C-Spine?[2] — YES → • C-Spine clear / • D/C collar

NO ↓

Cooperative: AP/Latera/Odontoid X-rays
Uncooperative: AP/Lateral X-rays

↓

Neurologic Exam — ABNORMAL → • Leave collar on[3] / • MRI / • Consider CT of C-Spine / • Consult Spine Service

NORMAL ↓

Normal and Adequate X-ray? — ABNORMAL → CT C-Spine

CT C-Spine — ABNORMAL → • Leave collar on[3] / • Consult Spine Service

NORMAL ↓ / NORMAL ↓

> 8 years   ≤ 8 years

≤ 8 years ↓ — Planning Head CT? — NO →

Planning Head CT? — YES ↓ — CT Head and C1-3 — ABNORMAL → • Leave collar on[3] / • Consult Spine Service

CT Head and C1-3 — NORMAL → Re-examine

Re-examine — NORMAL → • C-Spine clear / • D/C collar

Re-examine — ABNORMAL NEUROLOGIC EXAM → • Leave collar on[3] / • MRI / • Consider CT of C-Spine if not already done / • Consult Spine Service

ABNORMAL EXAM: C-SPINE TENDERNESS →

• Consider Flexion/Extension X-rays / • Consider Consult Spine Service

ABNORMAL OR INADEQUATE X-RAYS → • Leave collar on[3] / • Consider MRI

NORMAL AND ADEQUATE X-RAYS → • May discharge with close follow-up and consider removal of collar

[1] Awake and alert with GCS - 15
[2] Meets NEXUS criteria AND moves head in flexion/extension AND rotate 45 degrees to both sides with no pain.
[3] Change to long term cervicol spine collar as soon as appropriate.

FIGURE 2.1. Trauma Association of Canada (TAC) National Pediatric C-Spine Evaluation Pathway.

If a patient scenario does not have any of these features, it is highly unlikely that a cervical spine injury has been sustained; no cervical spine imaging is required. The child in this scenario has neck pain (midline) after a high risk mechanism. Imaging is needed, but what kind(s)?

Image Modality

Once the decision has been made to pursue cervical imaging, the next question is what modality is most efficacious and carries the least amount of risk to the patient. Unlike in suspected adult cervical injury, the potential side effects that radiation can carry in children creates the need to discriminate between scenarios that require CT imaging and those where plain films are adequate.

- *Plain radiographs*
  "Plain film" x-rays are almost always the first-line imaging choice to evaluate the cervical spine in neurologically intact children and those without significant obvious bony disruptions on exam.[10] When images include a lateral film combined with two orthogonal AP and odontoid views, the sensitivity for fracture detection is as high as 90%.[11] However, adequate films require several parameters be met. Visualization of C1–T1 is necessary. Without visualization to T1, the cervical spine fracture cannot be ruled out and cross-sectional imaging is necessary.
  Despite these potential challenges, plain films are the optimal initial imaging in nearly all cases of potential cervical spine trauma. *Start with radiographs prior to CT scan in all traumatic cases other than cases with a new neurologic defect, or possibly those children where a CT head is already being obtained to evaluate head trauma and cervical injury is suspected as well.* Initial radiographs should include lateral, AP, and odontoid views to maximize chances for identification of any abnormalities. The child in this scenario should initially receive plain film images in the ED to evaluate his cervical spine.
- *CT*
  As in adults, both the sensitivity and specificity of CT scan for identifying cervical spine fractures is approximately 98%. It remains the most successful test in diagnosing cervical spine fractures over all other image modalities. However, the radiation to which a CT scan exposes a patient is much more clinically significant in a child than an adult. A CT scan delivers approximately 1.5 times the dose of radiation to the spine compared to plain films. Further, the thyroid and skin are exposed

to upward of 15% more radiation from a CT of the cervical spine. Radiation exposure has a much higher propensity to cause cancers in children, and has been shown to increase the lifetime malignancy mortality risk by a significant percentage compared to adults.[12,13] Therefore, CT should not be used as the standard initial cervical imaging for most pediatric patients. However, in many cases CT can be used to further evaluate a fracture or other bony abnormality once visualized on radiographs. This is necessary for determining the extent of fractures, degrees of malunion, and accurate measurements of dislocations, and will often determine surgical course and planning.

CT scan should be reserved for any patient who has a suspicious or obviously abnormal finding on plain film, for those patients requiring imaging but for whom plain films are not achieving adequate visualization, or (as primary imaging INSTEAD OF radiographs) for those patients whose clinical picture likely already guarantees necessary exposure to CT scan radiation, namely, altered mental status, focal neurological defects, or obvious bony injury on exam.

- *MRI*

    There are instances in which neither x-ray nor CT scan are considered sufficient imaging modalities. In these select cases, MRI is necessary to evaluate for occult spinal injury. Pediatric patients are at a much higher risk of spinal cord injury without radiographic abnormality (SCIWORA) than are adults. This is due to ligamentous elasticity and bony anatomy allowing for hypermobility of the cervical spine.[14] As a result, MRI imaging should be performed on any pediatric patient who is displaying concerning neurologic deficits/abnormalities or has a significantly concerning neck exam, but has normal plain films and/or CT. This recommendation applies even to situations of reported transient focal neurologic deficits, who then had normal neurological exams once evaluated by a physician. This also applies to cases of persistent altered mental status after several reassessments without any additional focal neurological deficits.

    The MRI is unparalleled in its ability to evaluate for soft tissue injury, ligamentous injury, and damage to the spinal cord itself far better than a CT scan.[15] However, the test is not perfect, and has several downsides. It is much less successful than CT in detecting bony abnormalities or fractures. It is also an extremely time-consuming study to perform, occasionally necessitating significant sedation prior to pediatric patients receiving the scan. This can raise both cost and adverse outcomes. Finally, the test is simply not as readily available in many facilities.

As a rule, any child with an abnormal neurological exam, whether initially or after re-examination, will likely require both MRI and cervical CT-scan; order both of these studies on any patient with focal neurological deficits on exam. Furthermore, in children who are victims of significant trauma where cervical spine injuries are noted on imaging, additional imaging of the thoracolumbar spine is also indicated. If no pain or abnormalities are present on exam, plain films are adequate; however, in the presence of any suspicion of additional lower spine injury in setting of known cervical vertebral disruption, CT imaging of the thoracolumbar column is recommended.

CASE CONCLUSION

The child in the scenario had plain films that were suspicious for a fracture. A CT scan showed a stable cervical spine fracture. The thoracic and lumbar spine films were normal. The child was admitted to the neurosurgical service for definitive care.

KEY POINTS TO REMEMBER

- *In the setting of a child with a GCS of 15 and without a history of disease predisposing one to cervical spine injuries, the cervical spine can be cleared without imaging if the child has a normal neurological exam and normal neck exam.*
- *In the setting of an abnormal neurological exam, the cervical spine cannot be cleared without imaging; both CT and MRI are likely to be required by the spinal consult team.*

- In the setting of a normal neuro exam but abnormal neck exam with abnormal cervical spine radiographs, a CT scan of the cervical spine becomes necessary along with a spine consult for further workup.
- In the setting of a normal neuro exam, abnormal neck exam with normal cervical spine radiographs the physician must use their clinical judgment to determine whether the cervical exam is concerning enough to warrant additional imaging. Re-examination is key in this setting, as an improving physical exam is a sign that no additional imaging is indicated. A caveat to this is *if the patient is <8 years old and will require a head CT (due to head trauma, hematoma, etc.),when it is recommended to obtain C1–C3 CT imaging if the cervical spine cannot be initially cleared, even if initial x-rays are normal.*[16]
- In any instance where abnormalities are detected on imaging, or for whatever reason a cervical spine cannot be cleared, the patient is to remain in their C-collar, and the spine team is to be consulted for further evaluation and workup.

Further Reading

1. Patel JC, Tepas JJ 3rd, Mollitt DL, Pieper P. Pediatric cervical spine injuries: defining the disease. *J Pediatr Surg.* 2001;36:373.
2. Peclet MH, Newman KD, Eichelberger MR, et al. Patterns of injury in children. *J Pediatr Surg.* 1990;25:85.
3. Leonard JR, Jaffe DM, Kuppermann N, et al. Cervical spine injury patterns in children. *Pediatrics.* 2014;133:e1179.
4. EMS management of patients with potential spinal injury. *Ann Emerg Med.* 2015;66:445.
5. Curran C, Dietrich AM, Bowman MJ, et al. Pediatric cervical-spine immobilization: achieving neutral position? *J Trauma.* 1995;39:729.
6. EMS spinal precautions and the use of the long backboard. *Prehosp Emerg Care.* 2013;17:392.
7. Leonard JC, Kuppermann N, Olsen C, et al. Factors associated with cervical spine injury in children after blunt trauma. *Ann Emerg Med.* 2011;58:145.
8. Slaar A, Fockens MM, Wang J, et al. Triage tools for detecting cervical spine injury in pediatric trauma patients. *Cochrane Database Syst Rev.* 2017;12:CD011686.

9. Ehrlich PF, Wee C, Drongowski R, Rana AR. Canadian c-spine rule and the National Emergency X-Radiography Utilization Low-Risk Criteria for c-spine radiography in young trauma patients. *J Pediatr Surg.* 2009;44:987.

10. Chung S, Mikrogianakis A, Wales PW, et al. Trauma association of Canada Pediatric Subcommittee National Pediatric Cervical Spine Evaluation Pathway: consensus guidelines. *J Trauma.* 2011;70:873.

11. Cui LW, Probst MA, Hoffman JR, Mower WR. Sensitivity of plain radiography for pediatric cervical spine injury. *Emerg Radiol.* 2016;23:443.

12. Adelgais KM, Grossman DC, Langer SG, Mann FA. Use of helical computed tomography for imaging the pediatric cervical spine. *Acad Emerg Med.* 2004;11:228.

13. Rybicki F, Nawfel RD, Judy PF, et al. Skin and thyroid dosimetry in cervical spine screening: two methods for evaluation and a comparison between a helical CT and radiographic trauma series. *AJR Am J Roentgenol.* 2002;179:933.

14. Pang D. Spinal cord injury without radiographic abnormality in children, 2 decades later. *Neurosurgery.* 2004;55:1325.

15. Levitt MA, Flanders AE. Diagnostic capabilities of magnetic resonance imaging and computed tomography in acute cervical spinal column injury. *Am J Emerg Med.* 1991;9:131.

16. Chung S, Mikrogianakis A, Wales PW, et al. Trauma Association of Canada Pediatric Subcommittee National Pediatric Cervical Spine Evaluation Pathway: consensus guidelines. *J Trauma.* 2011;70:873.

3 Out and Out It Goes . . . Where It Stops . . . Who Knows

Danny Lammers, Christopher Marenco, Woo Do, and John Horton

A 2-year-old boy, with no medical problems, presents to the emergency department following an unwitnessed fall down stairs. He was found at the bottom of stairs and was initially inconsolable. He initially complained of pain to his mid abdomen, and has become increasingly somnolent over the past hour. On arrival to the pediatric trauma bay, the patient is noted to be minimally responsive. He is intubated with a pediatric endotracheal tube due to his altered mental status. Bilateral breath sounds are present and he is noted to be tachycardic with a heart rate of 155 beats per minute. Otherwise, the child's abdomen is noted to be tense and distended and his extremities are cool and mottled. He does not display any further external signs of trauma. Intravenous (IV) access is unable to be obtained, and therefore intraosseous (IO) access is placed. An E-FAST is performed which is concerning for a dark stripe in the splenorenal fossa.

What do you do now?

DISCUSSION

Within the United States, pediatric trauma is the leading cause of death among children and adolescents.[1] Traumatic injuries, both unintentional and intentional, represent a significant proportion of the emergency department visits within the pediatric population.[2] Due to differences in body surface area and physiologic response, pediatric trauma differs significantly from its adult counterpart. A thorough understanding of these differences remains crucial in the assessment and management of pediatric trauma patients. Alterations of normal vital signs for each age group remain a key piece of information that must not be forgotten in the trauma patient. Early recognition of vital sign abnormalities (tachycardia) and perfusion status (delayed capillary refill) can help to rapidly identify even subtle signs of shock. Hypotension is a late sign of shock, unlike adults, so a normal blood pressure does not exclude shock.

Initial trauma management relies on the rapid assessment of the presenting injury pattern, prioritization of any critical interventions necessary, appropriate resuscitation, and overall stabilization. This process should be initiated through an algorithmic approach defined by the primary survey as outlined within the Advanced Trauma Life Support (ATLS) guidelines (Figure 3.1). A stepwise, linear assessment of the airway, breathing and ventilation, circulation with hemorrhage control, evaluation of neurologic status, and complete exposure of the patient to ensure complete visualization simplifies and facilitates rapid assessment and management. This stepwise approach is the backbone of the ATLS algorithm. As with adults, any life-threatening conditions must be addressed at this point.[3]

Following stabilization of the child's airway and breathing, the circulatory status of the child should be assessed. The initial presentation of hemorrhagic shock is typically tachycardia following significant blood loss. Due to augmentation of their cardiac output via tachycardic compensation, as well as their robust vasoconstrictive response to hypovolemia, hypotension tends to be a late finding in shock in children. Current practice suggests blood pressure can be maintained among children with up to 45% blood loss.[3] However, their ability to tolerate shock once it clinically develops is diminished, adding to the importance of a high degree of suspicion for clinicians. Clinical dogma commonly teaches that the cool pediatric trauma

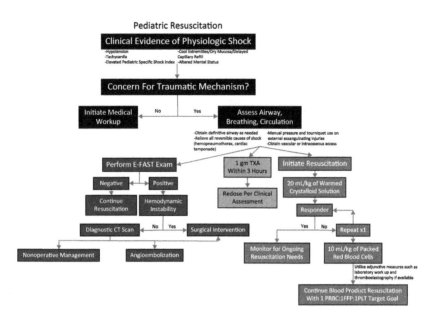

FIGURE 3.1. Pediatric rescucitation algorithm.

patient who is tachycardic beyond normal age-adjusted parameters should be considered in shock until proven otherwise. Other parameters to aid in the assessment for hypovolemic shock include a narrowed pulse pressure, altered consciousness, delayed capillary refill, and mottling of skin.[3] Finally, an elevated pediatric-specific shock index (SIPA), defined as heart rate/systolic blood pressure with cutoff values of SIPA >1.22 for ages 4–6, >1.0 (ages 7–12), and >0.9 (ages 13 and above), has demonstrated an increased need for transfusion and mortality among certain pediatric trauma populations.[4]

Once shock is suspected, initial inspection and physical exam of the patient can help elucidate the potential causes. As with adult trauma patients, major areas of concern include external bleeding, chest trauma resulting in pneumothorax, hemothorax, or cardiac tamponade, evidence of peritonitis or abdominal distension to suggest noncompressible intra-abdominal hemorrhage, pelvic instability, extremity fractures, or concern for spinal cord injury.

Search the patient for sources of external hemorrhage. If external sources of bleeding are identified, immediate source control should be initiated if amenable. Direct manual pressure is regarded as the first line of defense. The goal is to proximally compress the exsanguinating vessel to occlude blood flow. As of 2018, the Pediatric Trauma Society supports the use of tourniquets in the prehospital setting and during active resuscitation for exsanguinating hemorrhage in extremity trauma. Blind placement of clamps within hemorrhagic wounds should be avoided as the close proximity of principal nerves to the vascular structures places children at severe risk for permanent nerve damage. Long bone fractures should be reduced by the appropriate providers as this may further aid in hemostasis at the associated site of injury. Pediatric sized pelvic binders should also be placed over the greater trochanters within the trauma bay to reduce the pelvic volume in patients with concern for pelvic fracture. Should the patient initially present or become hemodynamically unstable during the initial evaluation, emergent surgical consultation and preparation for operative intervention is warranted.[5]

Replacement of exsanguinated volume is critical to reestablish and maintain hemodynamic stability. During the primary survey, IV access should be rapidly obtained. Catheter size may vary by age, however as a general rule one should place the largest catheter that can be reliably inserted, with multiple peripheral IV catheters being generally preferred. After three failed attempts at IV access, in a child in shock, use of IO access in a nonfractured extremity provides a rapid and safe alternative. Once access is achieved, both crystalloid and blood product administration can be safely performed via both IV and IO routes. Central venous access may be performed but should not delay initial attempts at rapid IV or IO access.[3,6]

Following IV or IO access, an initial fluid bolus of 20 mL/kg of warmed crystalloid solution, either lactated ringers or normal saline, should be initiated for the patient in suspected shock. Two crystalloid boluses (20 mL/kg) should be given prior to blood product administration. Should the initial two crystalloid boluses prove unsuccessful at correcting shock, compensated (normal blood pressure) or decompensated shock (hypotension), blood transfusion at 10mL/kg of packed red blood cells (PRBC) should be initiated. However, total transfusion volume should not exceed 1 unit per transfusion.[3] Despite poorly studied data within the pediatric trauma literature, blood product administration in many major trauma centers has evolved to use thromboelastography (TEG), which can provide a real-time functional measure of a patient's coagulation status. This allows for correction of specific coagulation deficits through the administration of fresh frozen plasma (FFP), cryoprecipitate, platelets (PLT), or tranexamic acid (TXA). However, mirroring standards within the adult population, a balanced ratio of 1 PRBC:1 FFP:1 PLT still remains a reasonable approach to blood product administration for the injured child due to the paucity of data surrounding TEG-based approaches. That being said, the pediatric trauma literature does not show a clear survival benefit to this balanced approach to component resuscitation.[3]

Studies have defined a transfusion threshold of 40mL/kg for all blood products administered in the first 24 hours as the optimal definition for massive transfusion in children.[7] This level has been shown to demarcate an increased risk for early and in-hospital death.[8] Realization of this threshold is typically a retrospective event thus, a massive transfusion protocol (MTP) is often initiated clinically when there is an anticipated need to replace greater than 50% of blood volume in 3 hours, 100% blood volume over the first 24 hours, or ongoing blood loss of greater than 10% of blood volume per minute.[9] Recent data suggests the mortality rate after development of shock, defined as hypotension or need for emergent blood in the trauma bay, to be disproportionally high; 46% of hypotensive patients, 42% of patients receiving transfusion, and 63% of hypotensive patients who received transfusions ultimately died.[10]

Permissive hypotensive resuscitation is a concept used in adult trauma to allow perfusion of vital organs while limiting ongoing blood loss by preventing the disturbance of an evolving clot. This concept has not been well researched in children and no current data support its use. In fact, high rates of concomitant traumatic brain injury in this population argue against permissive hypotension, as perfusion pressure to the brain would become limited.[11] Due to the altered physiologic response of the pediatric patient compared to the adult trauma patient, permissive hypotension is felt to be inappropriate by most pediatric trauma centers.

Regarding laboratory evaluation of the traumatically injured pediatric patient, it is crucial that a blood type and cross be sent with initial laboratory tests to ensure appropriately cross-matched blood products are being used. Serial assessment of hematocrit levels allows for identification of ongoing, especially occult, blood loss. Further labs of value on presentation and throughout resuscitation include BUN to assess for uremia, which may result in platelet dysfunction; creatinine, which may indicate renal injury secondary to malperfusion/hypoperfusion; coagulation panel, which can allude to evidence of trauma-induced coagulopathy and need for coagulation factors; fibrinogen levels to assess for fibrinogen consumption; lactate to assess for hypoperfusion; arterial blood gas to evaluate for acidosis; and base deficit further suggestive of malperfusion.

As with the adult trauma population, trauma-induced coagulopathy remains a complicating issue resulting in increased morbidity and mortality. As previously mentioned, TEG has been identified as a useful tool to assess coagulopathy in children and may be used if available. However, again, no data currently exits to support its use to guide resuscitative efforts. Conversely, an INR greater than 1.3 at admission and also at 24 hours was found to be associated with significantly increased mortality and acted as a marker for systemic dysregulation; however, INR should not be used as a target for coagulopathy correction.[12] Data from the previously stated study by Leeper et al., supports the sentiment that further work with TEG-based resuscitation in the pediatric population should be investigated.

Current practices in adult trauma, backed by the large prospective, international, multi-institution CRASH-2 trial, advocate for early, protocoled use of TXA in certain trauma cohorts. This practice was assessed in the pediatric trauma population and was found to be independently associated with decreased mortality and no adverse safety or medication-related complications when 1 gram of TXA was given within 3 hours of injury with the option to redose based on the assessment of the medical team.[13] While retrospective data indicates the use of TXA in pediatric patients with traumatic brain injury (TBI) is associated with improved neurologic outcomes,[14] the CRASH-3 trial is currently enrolling patients and should provide more insight into TXA use in TBI patients.[15] This remains an important concept to keep in mind as early protocolized TXA use continues to be debated among adult trauma surgery providers due to recent literature indicating a wide array of trauma-induced coagulopathy phenotypes based on TEG readings that suggest roughly one-third of patients display a phenotypic pattern that would not benefit from routine TXA use.[16] While there is no data to support this in the pediatric literature, TEG-guided resuscitation may allow for selective use of TXA for pediatric trauma patients.

CASE CONCLUSION

Due to concerns for hemorrhagic shock secondary to intra-abdominal bleeding based on the patient's clinical presentation and positive E-FAST, the patient was taken to the operating room for surgical exploration. While preparing to transfer the child to the operating room, laboratory studies were obtained and two 20 mL/kg fluid boluses of normal saline were administered. The child received 10 mL/kg of PRBCs in the operating room. Due to the unstable nature of the child, a CT scan was not pursued. An exploratory laparotomy was performed where a grade IV splenic injury was noted by a laceration of the hilar vessels at the inferior splenic pole, and a splenectomy was performed. The patient was transferred to the pediatric intensive care unit for postoperative management and he was successfully extubated the morning of postoperative day 1. He was transferred to the pediatric floor on postoperative day 3 and was discharged on postoperative day 5, following an uneventful hospital course. He was seen in clinic on postoperative day 15 and was administered vaccines against *Streptococcus pneumoniae*, *Haemophilus influenza*, and *Neisseria meningitidis* to protect against overwhelming postsplenectomy infection syndrome.

KEY POINTS TO REMEMBER

· Pediatric trauma resuscitation does not precisely mirror practices seen within the adult population. Differences in anatomy and physiologic response to acute blood loss directly alter the resuscitative management.
· While warmed crystalloid boluses are often initiated, early use of blood transfusion is recommended for those nonresponsive to crystalloid or with ongoing blood loss.
· Standard of care currently targets a 1PRBC:1FFP:1PLT goal.
· Though not yet standard of care, TEG-based resuscitative efforts are gaining popularity.
· Early TXA in the pediatric trauma patient in hemorrhagic shock is currently supported by the literature.
· Permissive hypotension should be avoided within pediatric cohorts.

Further Reading

1. Centers for Disease Control and Prevention. *10 Leading Causes of Death by Age Group, United States—2013*. Atlanta, GA: National Center for Injury Prevention and Control, Centers for Disease Control and Prevention; 2013.

2. Wier LM, Hao Y, Owens P, Washington R. *Overview of Children in the emergency department, 2010*. HCUP Statistical Brief #157. June 2013. Agency for Healthcare Research and Quality, Rockville, MD. http://www.hcup-us.ahrq.gov/reports/statbriefs/sb157.pdf

3. American College of Surgeons Committee on Trauma. *Advanced Trauma Life Support (ATLS) Student Course Manual*. 9th ed. Chicago: American College of Surgeons; 2012.

4. Acker SN, et al. Shock index, pediatric age-adjusted (SIPA) is more accurate than age-adjusted hypotension for trauma team activation. *Surgery*. 2017;161(3): 803–7.

5. Cunningham A, Auerbach M, Cicero M, Jafri M. Tourniquet usage in prehospital care and resuscitation of pediatric trauma patients—Pediatric Trauma Society position statement. *J Trauma Acute Care Surg*. 2018;85(4):665.

6. Stafford PW, Blinman TA, Nance ML. Practical points in evaluation and resuscitation of the injured child. *Surg Clin North Am*. 2002;82(2):273.

7. Horst J, Leonard JC, Vogel R, Jacobs R, Spinella PC. A survey of US and Canadian hospitals' paediatric massive transfusion protocol policies. *Transfus Med*. 2016;26:49–56.

8. Neff LP, Cannon JW, Morrison JJ, et al. Clearly defining pediatric massive transfusion: cutting through the fog and friction with combat data. *J Trauma Acute Care Surg*. 2015;78:22–8.

9. Diab YA, Wong EC, Luban NL. Massive transfusion in children and neonates. *Br J Haematol*. 2013;161(1):15–26.

10. Leeper, CM, Mckenna, C, Gaines, BA. Too little too late: hypotension and blood transfusion in the trauma bay are independent predictors of death in injured children. *J Trauma Acute Care Surg*. 2018;85(4):674–8.

11. Schneier AJ, Shields BJ, Hostetler SG, et al. Incidence of pediatric traumatic brain injury and associated hospital resource utilization in the United States. *Pediatrics*. 2006;118:483–92.

12. Leeper CM, Kutcher M, McKenna C, et al. Acute traumatic coagulopathy in a critically injured pediatric population: definition, trend over time, and outcomes. *J Trauma Acute Care Surg*. 2016;81(1):34–41.

13. Shakur H, Roberts I, Bautista R, et al. Effects of tranexamic acid on death, vascular occlusive events, and blood transfusion in trauma patients with significant haemorrhage (CRASH-2): a randomised, placebo-controlled trial. *Lancet*. 2010;376(9734):23–32.

14. Eckert MJ, Wertin TM, Tyner SD, Nelson DW, Izenberg S, Martin MJ. Tranexamic acid administration to pediatric trauma patients in a combat setting: the pediatric

trauma and tranexamic acid study (PED-TRAX). *J Trauma Acute Care Surg*. 2014;77(6):852–8.

15. Dewan Y, Komolafe EO, Megia-Mantilla JH, Perel P, Roberts I, Shakur H. CRASH-3—tranexamic acid for the treatment of significant traumatic brain injury: study protocol for an international randomized, double-blind, placebo-controlled trial. *Trials*. 2012;13:87.

16. Moore EE, Moore HB, Gonzalez E, Chapman M, Hansen KC, Sauaia A, Sillman CC, Banerjee A. Postinjury fibrinolysis shutdown: rationale for selective tranexamic acid. *J Trauma Acute Care Surg*. 2015;78(601000006): S65–9.

4 A Tumble for a Cookie

Nancy Rixe

A mother presents with her 2-year-old son who, 2 hours ago, fell while climbing onto a stool 2 feet off the ground, striking his head on the linoleum floor. His mother said that he cried immediately and did not appear to lose consciousness, but is more irritable and is crying more than usual. He slept throughout the car ride over, which is unusual for him, and has had 1 episode of nonbilious, non-bloody emesis. Upon initial assessment, his temperature is 37.2°C, heart rate is 115 bpm, blood pressure is 90/62 mmHg, respiratory rate is 18 breaths per minute, and the oxygen saturation is 99% in room air. He appears alert and calm in his mother's arms, with no bruising, hematomas, or step-offs of the scalp. His extraocular muscle movements are intact, and he easily reaches for objects with both hands. His heart sounds are regular without murmur and his lungs are clear. His abdominal, back, and extremity exams are normal. He cries when he is put down but walks without difficulty. His mother is worried that he has a serious brain injury.

What do you do now?

MINOR TRAUMATIC BRAIN INJURY

Discussion

Traumatic brain injury (TBI) in children causes significant morbidity and accounts for over 3,000 pediatric deaths per year.[1] The mechanism of pediatric TBI varies by age such that young children more frequently incur head injury from falls or nonaccidental trauma, while older children are more subject to head injury following motor-vehicle accidents.[2] Minor head injury, defined by a Glasgow Coma Score (GCS) of greater than or equal to 14, is the most commonly encountered type of pediatric head trauma in the emergency department (ED).[3] Following minor head injury, children may present with variable signs and symptoms depending on their age, physiology, and developmental stage. A key part of caring for children after minor head injury includes an understanding of the pathophysiology of neurologic injury and how it contributes to a child's clinical presentation.

The brain is suspended in cerebrospinal fluid (CSF) and encased within the calvarium, which, after 2 years of age, becomes a fixed structure. Due to the rigid nature of the skull, perfusion of the brain relies on precise autoregulation to maintain cerebral perfusion pressure (CPP) such that CPP = mean arterial pressure (MAP) – intracranial pressure (ICP). In the setting of traumatic injury, one of the components within the calvarium (brain, CSF, or blood) may increase in volume, and, if not met by a reciprocal decrease in one of the remaining components, this will lead to an increase in ICP and a decrease in CPP.[2] If unmitigated, this imbalance can lead to brain herniation and death.

Symptoms of increased ICP and herniation can range from subtle to severe. In early infancy the cranial sutures remain open, allowing the intracranial space to expand. This expansion preserves CPP and mental status, while allowing for external signs of increasing ICP, including rapidly expanding head circumference, congested bridging scalp veins and a "sun downing" gaze. Older infants and children may present with nonspecific signs like vomiting, fatigue, and irritability. Ultimately, if the process continues, children may develop decreased level of consciousness, persistent vomiting, lethargy, difficulty walking, and somnolence. Vital signs aberrations that are indicative of imminent herniation include bradycardia, hypertension, and irregular respirations, also known as the Cushing Triad.[2]

While the signs and symptoms of severe intracranial injury (ICI) following major head injury* tend to be characteristic and more easily apparent, those following minor head injury present more of a diagnostic challenge to clinicians. For example, vomiting is a very common event following a minor head injury and, in isolation, is not necessarily indicative of intracranial pathology.[2,4] Conversely, irritability in an infant following an apparently minor head injury may be the only indication of serious ICI. Therefore, it is important to tailor one's assessment following minor head injury to the age and developmental stage of each patient. Verbal children should be asked about headache, neck pain, paresthesias, weakness, and amnesia. Preverbal or nonverbal children should be assessed for change in behavior, irritability, persistent vomiting, or change in level of consciousness. All children, regardless of age or ability to communicate, should undergo a thorough assessment of the traumatic mechanism, including, when appropriate, height of the fall, surface impacted, velocity of striking object, speed of the vehicle, presence or absence of appropriate restraints (car seat, booster seat, seat belt), extrusion or intrusion of the vehicle compartments and status of the other passengers. In addition, predisposing factors that may have contributed to the traumatic event should be elicited from the patient, caregiver, or witness(es), including seizure disorder, medications, bleeding or clotting disorders, known or suspected arrhythmia, and drug or alcohol intake.[2] These historical clues provide an important context for the physical exam, the findings of which can be subtle or even normal in the setting of ICI.

All children presenting after a traumatic injury should have a rapid primary assessment of airway, breathing, and circulation. In the setting of known or suspected head injury, a focused secondary assessment should include calculation of Glasgow Coma Scale (GCS), which assigns a score to eye opening, verbal function, and motor function and can range from the lowest score of 3 to the highest score of 15.[2] Importantly, the modified GCS for preverbal children has been shown to have similar utility to the standard GCS for older children and adults.[5] Despite this, it is important to remember that a normal GCS does not preclude serious ICI. For example, a

---

* Major head injury refers to those children who are not considered low risk, including those who present with, i.e., GCS < 14, altered mental status, and palpable skull fracture.

child with an epidural hematoma, or a collection of blood between the dura and the skull, may classically experience a "lucid interval," during which their neurologic exam is completely normal despite rapidly expanding and potentially life-threatening intracranial bleeding.[2] Thus, the clinician, even in the setting of a well-appearing child with a normal GCS, should thoroughly evaluate all children following head injury.

In addition, all children who have experienced head trauma should have a detailed physical exam including close inspection of the head, neck, and trunk for external signs of trauma. A complete neurologic exam should also be performed, including assessment of mental status, cranial nerves, sensation, motor function, reflexes, cerebellar function, assessment of gait, and observation of developmentally appropriate tasks. Specific findings that are potentially indicative of ICI include a bulging fontanelle, palpable skull fracture, periorbital or postauricular hematoma, clear fluid from the nose or ears, papilledema, and retinal hemorrhage.[2] The constellation of findings on history and physical exam are paramount in determining the appropriate work-up of children presenting with head injury.

Types of head injury depend on the structures involved. Head injury can be incurred by the scalp, skull, intracranial contents, or a combination of all three. Injuries to the scalp include lacerations, contusions, and hematomas. While these injuries may appear to be superficial and inconsequential, they may also signify injury to deeper structures. For example, a subgaleal hematoma occurs when deep vessels within the scalp are torn and bleed between the galea and periosteum, an injury that requires more force than a simple laceration or contusion.[2]

Similarly, injuries to the skull may be a harbinger of underlying ICI, particularly in infants. Depressed skull fractures, defined as a fracture that displaces the inner table of the skull by more than the thickness of the bone itself, are often palpable on exam and warrant further workup given the force that is necessary to create them.[2,6] Basilar skull fractures carry a high risk of ICI in children and classically present with CSF otorrhea or rhinorrhea, periorbital swelling, and postauricular swelling.[2]

Intracranial injuries can be divided into focal and diffuse. Focal injuries can be localized to a particular area of the brain and include contusions, hematomas, and penetrating injuries. Diffuse injuries refer to those that involve the majority of the intracranial contents and may not be readily apparent on initial imaging, including diffuse axonal injury and diffuse brain swelling.[2] Children with injury to the intracranial contents may not have obvious injury to external structures; thus, clinicians must have a diagnostic framework available to appropriately evaluate children with potential ICI.

Cranial computed tomography (CT) is the diagnostic imaging modality of choice for identifying ICI in children presenting with head trauma. However, CT uses ionizing radiation, which has been associated with a 1 in 1,000 risk of lethal malignancies in children.[7] Furthermore, less than 10% of children presenting after minor TBI have TBI identified on CT, and far fewer require neurosurgical intervention.[3] For this reason, it is imperative to practice judicious use of cranial CT when evaluating children presenting with head trauma. The Pediatric Emergency Care Applied Research Network (PECARN) prospectively derived and validated a clinical prediction rule to identify children at very low risk of clinically important (ci) TBI after blunt head trauma in whom CT may be unnecessary (Figure 4.1).[2] The algorithm includes age, GCS, signs of altered mental status, mechanism of injury, loss of consciousness greater than 5 seconds, abnormal behavior, and presence of palpable skull fracture and nonfrontal scalp hematoma. Over 40,000 children younger than 18 years presenting to 25 PECARN-affiliated North American EDs with head injury were evaluated and included in the derivation cohort. Clinically important TBI was identified in 0.9% of patients, while neurosurgery was performed in only 0.1% of patients. For children under 2 years of age with no PECARN risk criteria, the prediction rule had a sensitivity of 100% (95% CI 86.3–100) with negative predictive value of 100% (95% CI 99.7–100) for ruling out ciTBI.[3,8] For children > 2 years of age with no PECARN risk criteria, the prediction rule was 96% sensitive (95% CI 89.0–99.6) with negative predictive value of 99.95% (95% CI 99.8–99.99) for ruling out ciTBI.[3,8] While this prediction rule has started to guide the use of cranial CT for pediatric head trauma, it should not be applied to all children presenting to the ED with head injury. For example, children presenting with a GCS less than 14, palpable skull fracture, or change in mental status have a higher risk of ICI and should be evaluated with a cranial CT scan, regardless of other risk factors. Ultimately, the treating clinician should be aware of and comfortable with the prediction rules that exist and be able to apply them

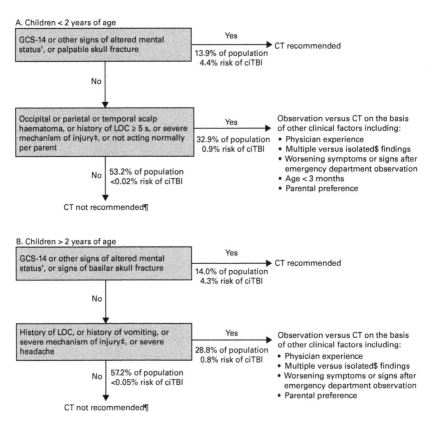

FIGURE 4.1. PECARN suggested CT algorithm for children presenting after minor head trauma.

Reprinted from The Lancet, 3:374, Kuppermann N et al, Identification of children at very low risk of clinically-important brain injuries after head trauma: a prospective cohort study, 1160-70, Copyright 2009, with permission from Elsevier.

correctly within each clinical context in order to properly diagnose and treat children with traumatic head injury.

The treatment and prognosis of pediatric head trauma depend entirely on the injuries identified during evaluation. Patients in whom ICI is identified, regardless of symptoms, should undergo neurosurgical evaluation and close monitoring. Asymptomatic or minimally symptomatic patients who met PECARN low risk criteria can be safely observed in the ED and, in the absence of changing signs or symptoms, can be safely discharged home with primary care follow-up.[3]

CASE CONCLUSION

In the case of our patient, he had no further episodes of emesis and according to his parents, returned to his baseline mental status. In accordance with the PECARN prediction rule, he was discharged home after a 4-hour observation period and suffered no neurological sequelae.

KEY POINTS TO REMEMBER

· All children presenting with head trauma should undergo a comprehensive history with a focus on the mechanism of injury and predisposing risk factors for injury. A detailed physical exam, including age-appropriate GCS calculation, should be performed to assess for signs of basilar skull fracture (hemotympanum, CSF otorrhea, periorbital ecchymoses, posterior auricular ecchymoses), cervical spine injury, and neurological deficits.
· Signs of increased ICP present differently in infants and children; thus, clinicians must be aware of these differences in order to appropriately diagnose and manage minor head injury, particularly in the absence of a clear history of trauma.
· Clinical prediction rules have been created to assist clinicians in using CT scans to mitigate the risk of unnecessary cranial radiation while also minimizing the chance of missing a ciTBI in children. Clinicians must be aware of and comfortable with applying these rules correctly to pediatric patients with head trauma.
· Ultimately, it is important to practice shared decision-making with the parents and guardians in order to facilitate appropriate care of children presenting with head injury.

Further Reading

1. Centers for Disease Control and Prevention NCfIPaC. *TBI-Related Emergency Department Visits, Hospitalizations, and Deaths (EDHDs)*. https://www.cdc.gov/traumaticbraininjury/data/tbi-edhd.html. Updated March 29, 2019. Accessed May 6, 2019.

2. Schutzman S. Injury—head. In: G Fleisher, S Ludwig, eds. *Textbook of Pediatric Emergency Medicine*. 6th ed. Philadelphia, PA: Williams & Wilkins; 2010.

3. Kuppermann N, Holmes JF, Dayan PS, et al. Identification of children at very low risk of clinically-important brain injuries after head trauma: a prospective cohort study. *Lancet*. 2009;374(9696):1160–70.

4. Dayan PS, Holmes JF, Atabaki S, et al. Association of traumatic brain injuries with vomiting in children with blunt head trauma. *Ann Emerg Med*. 2014;63(6):657–65.

5. Borgialli DA, Mahajan P, Hoyle JD, et al. Performance of the pediatric Glasgow Coma Scale Score in the evaluation of children with blunt head trauma. *Acad Emerg Med*. 2016;23(8):878–84.

6. Greenes DS, Schutzman SA. Clinical indicators of intracranial injury in head-injured infants. *Pediatrics*. 1999;104(4 Pt 1):861–7.

7. Brenner D, Elliston C, Hall E, Berdon W. Estimated risks of radiation-induced fatal cancer from pediatric CT. *AJR Am J Roentgenol*. 2001;176(2):289–96.

8. Schonfeld D, Bressan S, Da Dalt L, Henien MN, Winnett JA, Nigrovic LE. Pediatric Emergency Care Applied Research Network head injury clinical prediction rules are reliable in practice. *Arch Dis Child*. 2014;99(5):427–31.

5   Down a Slippery Slope

Jennifer E. Melvin

A 5-year-old male presents to the emergency
department after colliding with a tree while downhill
sledding. He is complaining of chest pain. His
mother is present and states that the accident was
unwitnessed, but she found him crying near a
tree at the bottom of a hill. He is tearful on arrival,
with a heart rate of 162, blood pressure of 90/62,
respiratory rate of 44 and a pulse oximeter reading
of 97% on room air. His examination is notable for
mild swelling over the sternum and obvious pain
with palpation over his anterior chest wall; however,
no bruising, deformities or crepitus is appreciated.
He has clear breath sounds with good aeration on
bilateral auscultation. His cardiac and abdominal
examinations are benign. His Glasgow Coma Score is
14, with one point off for verbal responses. The rest of
his primary and secondary trauma assessments are
unremarkable. The patient is otherwise healthy and
fully immunized and, prior to this event, had been in
his usual state of health.

What do you do now?

DISCUSSION

Although trauma is a leading cause of morbidity and mortality in the pediatric population, pediatric chest trauma accounts for only a small percentage. In the United States, only approximately 5% of children who present to a pediatric trauma center have thoracic injuries. The reason for this low percentage is likely multifactorial; either the thoracic injury was sustained during such a severe mechanism that it was not survivable or there was a low-impact direct chest trauma that did not result in injury. Notably, pediatric patients are less susceptible than adults to certain torso injuries, such as rib fractures, as a result of the increased compliance of their chest wall.

Torso trauma in children is usually a result of extreme blunt force trauma, including falls, motor vehicle accidents, nonaccidental trauma, and assaults. Not surprisingly, these mechanisms rarely result in isolated chest wall injuries. More direct torso trauma may also be secondary to isolated blunt forces, such as those sustained in repetitive sports such as gymnastics or wrestling. Less commonly, torso trauma can result from penetrating trauma, such as gunshot or stab wounds.

The most common pediatric torso injuries include pneumothorax, hemothorax, pulmonary contusion, and rib fractures. Sternal fractures, scapular fractures, tracheal or esophageal injuries, large vessel injuries, and diaphragmatic injuries may also occur but are much less common. Blunt cardiac injury is atypical in the pediatric population but, if severe, often presents with arrhythmias or shock either prior to arrival or in the emergency department.

The patient in this scenario has sustained a direct, isolated trauma to his chest. In addition to the swelling and tenderness present on physical exam, he has notable tachycardia and tachypnea, which all together warrant a complete primary and secondary trauma assessment. Symptoms concerning for torso trauma include chest pain, shortness of breath, tachypnea, and/or hypoxia. Abnormal findings on examination of the chest wall, such as ecchymosis, swelling, lacerations, abrasions, pain with palpation, crepitus, abnormal breath sounds, or muffled heart tones, should raise suspicion for internal thoracic injuries. Agitation may also be a sign of hypoxia or pain. A threatened airway or difficulty breathing should be addressed immediately and prior to continuing with the remainder of the assessment. A thorough evaluation for abdominal injuries is warranted in patients with a thoracic injury given the close proximity of the abdominal and chest cavity contents. Particular care should also be given to patients with a low Glasgow Coma Score, intracranial hemorrhage, or multisystem injuries, particularly if there is a femur fracture present, as these patients often had a severe injury mechanism and are therefore at an increased risk for torso injury. Careful attention to vital signs is key to identifying associated injuries. In patients who present for chest trauma evaluation, the physical exam, in combination with an electrocardiogram and imaging tests, indicates whether resuscitative procedures, further evaluation, and/or treatment are warranted.

A chest radiograph and an electrocardiogram are appropriate initial screening tools for pediatric patients presenting after trauma with specific concern for torso injuries. Chest radiographs have a high sensitivity for the most common torso injuries, including pneumothorax, hemothorax, pneumomediastinum, and rib fractures. Although the anterioposterior (AP) chest radiograph view is routinely obtained in pediatric trauma patients, a lateral view chest radiograph is the diagnostic modality of choice for sternal fracture or sternal dislocation, as these injuries are usually present in the sagittal plane and therefore may be missed on the AP view. Notably, a retrospective case series found that only 47% of sternal fractures were identified on chest radiograph. However, further studies suggest that positive findings on chest radiographs may better predict clinically significant outcomes and that cases not initially visualized on imaging are less likely to require intervention. If there is persistent clinical concern for fracture despite a negative chest radiograph, ultrasound offers another imaging modality option. Ultrasonography has become an important part of the trauma evaluation, as it offers a quick bedside assessment of the heart, lungs, and abdomen. Although diagnostic ultrasounds are operator dependent, several recent studies have demonstrated its high sensitivity and specificity in diagnosing sternal fractures. A chest computed tomography (CT) may also be indicated for further evaluation if there remains concern for an unidentified or more serious underlying injury.

This patient underwent AP and lateral chest radiographs, which revealed an isolated sternal fracture (see Figure 5.1). Depending on the mechanism of injury, sternal fractures or sternal dislocations may be an isolated finding,

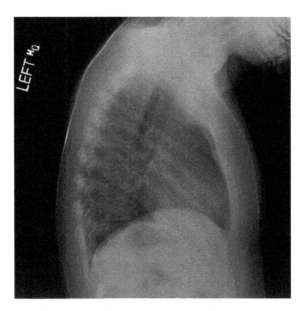

FIGURE 5.1. Lateral chest radiograph demonstrating a sternal fracture.

or they may serve as an indicator of other underlying injuries. Blunt cardiac injury, rib fracture, pulmonary contusion, pneumomediastinum, and aortic injury may be seen in conjunction with sternal fractures. Historically, blunt cardiac injury secondary to trauma has been associated with sternal fractures when the fracture results from a severe mechanism of injury; however, no clear association between depth of displacement of the fracture and cardiac injury has been described. Further laboratory data and imaging, such as an electrocardiogram (ECG), troponin levels, and an echocardiogram, may be warranted if there is concern for cardiac injury. This patient had an ECG, which was normal.

Rib fractures are most commonly identified on chest radiograph. Compared to displaced sternal fractures, multiple rib fractures correlate better with additional intrathoracic and/or intra-abdominal injuries. Therefore, especially when multiple rib fractures are present, further evaluation of both intrathoracic and intraabdominal cavity contents is essential. When assessing for pulmonary contusions, initial chest radiographs are often negative. Imaging with a chest CT is more sensitive for early detection of a pulmonary contusion than a chest radiograph, with 100% sensitivity for chest CT compared with only 47% sensitivity for an early chest radiograph. However, despite the higher sensitivity of a chest CT for pulmonary contusion, when considering its general utility in this patient population, several studies suggest that the incidence of clinically significant torso injuries, including thoracic aorta injury, is unusual; therefore, routine use of chest CT for screening purposes is not warranted. Nevertheless, chest CT with angiography may be specifically indicated in patients who have sustained a significant deceleration mechanism, especially if there is mediastinum widening or shift or aortic knob shift on chest radiograph, as these patients are at an increased risk for aortic injury.

The clinical course of pediatric patients presenting with chest trauma varies depending on the presence and severity of any associated injuries.

The patient in this scenario was diagnosed with an isolated sternal fracture on chest radiograph, with a normal ECG. In general, isolated sternal fractures resulting from low-impact mechanisms are associated with a good overall prognosis. The anatomy of the sternum comprises three main parts: the manubrium, the body, and the xiphoid process. Approximately 70% of sternal fractures involve the sternal body, and a transverse fracture through the midsternal body is the most common type of fracture. Most sternal fractures can be managed conservatively with supportive measures after a period of observation; however, surgical intervention may be required depending on the severity and displacement of the fracture. Specifically, open surgical reduction may be indicated for unstable or displaced fractures, especially if there is any compromise of cardiopulmonary function. If the sternal fracture is associated with other injuries, treatment plans may vary accordingly. Rib fractures usually do not require specific intervention unless they are multiple in number or a flail chest is present. Patients with rib fractures require adequate pain control to avoid decreased tidal volume and the associated increased risk of atelectasis and/or pneumonia. The treatment of a moderate-to-large or persistent pneumothorax or a hemothorax often includes drainage with chest tube thoracostomy. A tension pneumothorax with cardiopulmonary compromise can develop in up to 20% of pediatric patients after a simple pneumothorax and requires immediate needle decompression. Pulmonary contusions usually only require supportive measures; however, they can progress in the hours after injury and should therefore be monitored closely. When present, large vessel injuries require consultation with a pediatric thoracic surgeon. Recovery from an isolated sternal fracture often has a good prognosis, with the majority of patients achieving complete recovery. This patient was admitted for observation and received serial assessments. He did not develop any complications or require any operative interventions and was discharged home with close follow-up.

KEY POINTS TO REMEMBER

· Chest injuries in pediatric trauma patients are unusual but, when present, are often associated with other injuries.
· Chest radiographs are a good screening tool for pediatric chest trauma.
· Isolated sternal fractures often do not require intervention and have an overall good prognosis.

Further Reading
1. Berland M, Oger M, Cauchois E, Retornaz K, Arnoux V, Dubus JC. Pulmonary contusion after bumper car collision: case report and review of the literature. *Respir Med Case Rep.* 2018;25:293–5.
2. Clancy K, Velopulos C, Bilaniuk JW, et al. Screening for blunt cardiac injury: an Eastern Association for the Surgery of Trauma practice management guideline. *J Trauma Acute Care Surg.* 2012;73(5 Suppl 4):S301–6.
3. Ferguson LP, Wilkinson AG, Beattie TF. Fracture of the sternum in children. *Emerg Med J.* 2003;20(6):518–20.
4. Khoriati AA, Rajakulasingam R, Shah R. Sternal fractures and their management. *J Emerg Trauma Shock.* 2013;6(2):113–6.
5. Ramgopal S, Shaffiey SA, Conti KA. Pediatric sternal fractures from a Level 1 trauma center. *J Pediatr Surg.* 2018;54(8):1628–31.
6. Reynolds SL. Pediatric thoracic trauma: recognition and management. *Emerg Med Clin North Am.* 2018;36(2):473–83.
7. Tovar JA, Vazquez JJ. Management of chest trauma in children. *Paediatr Respir Rev.* 2013;14(2):86–91.

8. van As AB, Manganyi R, Brooks A. Treatment of thoracic trauma in children: literature review, Red Cross War Memorial Children's Hospital data analysis, and guidelines for management. *Eur J Pediatr Surg*. 2013;23(6):434–43.

9. Yanchar NL, Woo K, Brennan M, et al. Chest x-ray as a screening tool for blunt thoracic trauma in children. *J Trauma Acute Care Surg*. 2013;75(4):613–9.

10. You JS, Chung YE, Kim D, Park S, Chung SP. Role of sonography in the emergency room to diagnose sternal fractures. *J Clin Ultrasound*. 2010;38(3):135–7.

6 When Boo Boos Are Bad

Kaileen Jafari and Jessica J. Wall

A 7-year-old girl presents to your emergency department via ambulance after a high-speed motor vehicle collision. She was restrained in the back of the vehicle with a seatbelt. Medics report it was a head-on collision with a fatality, and your patient complained of some nausea and abdominal pain en route. On arrival, she has a temperature of 36.8°C, blood pressure of 90/60, heart rate of 130 bpm, and regular respirations of 20 bpm with an oxygen saturation of 98% on room air. She appears scared, but is alert and oriented. On your trauma survey you note an abrasion to the right forehead and tachycardia, and her abdomen has hypoactive bowel sounds with a linear bruise across the lower quadrants and mild diffuse tenderness. Palpation of the spine elicits tenderness in lower lumbar region without palpable step-offs. There are no are other obvious injuries on your exam.

What do you do next?

DISCUSSION

The Seatbelt Sign

The classic patterned abdominal finding, described as a linear abdominal bruise across the abdomen caused by a lap belt, is known as the seatbelt sign (see Figure 6.1). It was first reported in 1962 by Garrett et al., who found an association between abdominal wall bruising, internal abdominal injury and spinal fractures. Mechanistically, these injuries are thought to occur when the torso is hyperflexed over the 2-point restraint, resulting in compression of the abdominal contents and injury to the vertebrae and supporting structures of the spine.[1] Patients who are 4–9 years old are at particularly high risk for injuries secondary to lap-belt use, as their underdeveloped iliac crests do not provide sufficient anchoring for the lap belt. During a motor vehicle collision, upward slippage of the belt and subsequent compression of the abdomen may lead to abdominal and spinal injury. Children less than 8 years old or 80 pounds when restrained without a booster seat, and those children who improperly wear a 3-point restraint, are also at increased risk for this type of injury.

The blunt abdominal trauma associated with a seatbelt sign and/or significant mechanism can result in solid organ injury (e.g., liver, spleen, pancreas), hollow viscus injury (e.g., intestine, colon), and spinal injury or fracture. Recent data indicates the seatbelt sign specifically increases the likelihood of the hollow viscus injury when compared to children in motor vehicle accidents without this sign. Typical hollow viscus injuries include intestinal hematomas, contusion, seromuscular tears, or devascularization of the mesentery. Data from the largest population-based study on this subject found the seatbelt sign to have a high positive predictive value of 99.9%, with a number needed to treat of only 8.7.[2] Interestingly, children with a seatbelt sign and no abdominal pain or tenderness on examination still had a 5.7% risk of intra-abdominal injury, with only 2.2% requiring urgent surgical treatment.[3] This data suggests that conservative management is acceptable if the patient is hemodynamically stable and can be clinically observed with serial examinations.

When managing a pediatric patient with a seatbelt sign, the first question is, what is the best imaging choice? If available, a focused assessment with sonography in trauma (FAST exam) could be used as a

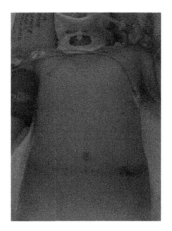

FIGURE 6.1. Seatbelt sign.

P. Raychaudhuri, N. K. Cheung, C. Bendinelli, M. Puvaneswary, R. Ferch, and Rajendra Kumar, "Seatbelt: A Double-Edged Sword," *Case Reports in Pediatrics*, vol. 2012, Article ID 326936, 3 pages, 2012. https://doi.org/10.1155/2012/326936.

screening tool to detect free intraperitoneal fluid, which if present in an otherwise stable patient, would indicate urgent need for computerized tomography (CT) of the abdomen and pelvis. However, even though a FAST exam with evidence of free intraperitoneal fluid would indicate need for further imaging in a hemodynamically stable patient, the sensitivity of this exam is insufficient to exclude need for further imaging if no free intraperitoneal fluid is detected. It is important to remember that the presence of a seatbelt sign is associated with a 232-fold increased risk of intra-abdominal injury compared to children with history of blunt trauma and absence of this sign.[2] Thus a CT of the abdomen and pelvis should be strongly considered.

Hollow viscus injuries secondary to abdominal trauma can be difficult to assess with imaging. Ultrasound has not been found to be sufficiently sensitive to detect hollow viscus injury and is not routinely used for this purpose. Computed tomography is frequently the diagnostic tool used in children presenting to the emergency department with concern for intra-abdominal injury. However, even high-resolution CT still has an imperfect sensitivity of 76%–98% for hollow viscus injury.[4,5] If not directly detected, other supportive CT findings such as mesenteric fat streaking, thickening of bowel wall, and intra-abdominal free air in the absence of solid organ injury can aid in the diagnosis of intestinal injury.

A seatbelt sign is also associated with spinal fractures, and requires either lateral lumbar plain film radiography (x-ray) or CT of the lumbar spine to evaluate for these potential injuries. Studies indicated that intra-abdominal injuries and spinal fractures co-occur in approximately 15% of patients.[2] The most frequent spinal fracture seen in patients with a seatbelt sign is a Chance fracture, which is an uncommon compression fracture of the anterior vertebral body combined with a transverse fracture that extends posteriorly. In one series, 43% of children with this fracture had a neurological deficit at the time of injury and only approximately half of these patients fully recovered.[6,7] This type of injury may also result in disruption of the posterior ligaments of the spine. Stepwise imaging of the spine is reasonable. Initial imaging may include lateral plain film radiographs followed by CT of the lumbar spine or MRI of the lumbar spine (any patient with a neurologic deficit or for evaluation of the posterior elements). Treatment options depend on the type of injury suffered. The presence of any neurologic deficits requires urgent surgical intervention, and those fractures which are significantly displaced or have a ligamentous injury often require a hyperextension brace or cast. Reassuringly, the majority of patients with Chance fractures have a good outcome without significant neurological defect.[1,2,7,8]

While the assessment and management of pediatric patients with blunt abdominal trauma and a seatbelt sign should be guided by history and exam, definitive imaging with a CT of the abdomen and pelvis verses prolonged observation with serial exams should be strongly considered. Laboratory assessment with a complete blood count, basic metabolic panel, liver function tests, lipase, and urinalysis should be obtained to evaluate for solid organ injury. Further, a type and screen should be obtained should blood products become necessary for resuscitation. Surgical consultation will be helpful in determining next steps for a patient with confirmed or suspected injury to the bowel or any other intra-abdominal organs. Free air in the abdomen and often other hollow viscus injury will require laparoscopy or laparotomy. Management of solid organ injury may be conservative management with serial exams versus operative depending on extent of solid organ damage, risk of further blood loss, hemodynamic stability, and associated injuries.

The Handlebar Sign

Another type of abdominal mark often associated with significant intra-abdominal injury is the Handlebar Sign (see Figure 6.2). This physical exam finding consists of a ring-shaped bruise on the abdomen secondary to direct impact from the exterior ends of a bicycle handlebar. This type of injury has the potential to cause significant intra-abdominal damage, as even at relatively low collision velocities the handlebar may transmit significant focal blunt force to the abdomen.[9,10] A wide variety of intra-abdominal injuries have been reported in association with handlebar injuries, including hollow viscus injury with rates of GI perforation of approximately 10%, and solid organ injuries occurring at rates between 20% and 37%.[11] Numerous other abdominal injuries have been reported following handlebar impact, including traumatic abdominal wall hernias and rupture, bile duct rupture, intestinal injury, abdominal aortic rupture, traumatic arterial occlusion, groin injury, and even death.[12,13]

The approach to a patient with a handlebar sign is similar to the patient with the seatbelt sign. Physical exam to assess for abdominal tenderness and laboratory exam including complete blood counts, basic metabolic panel,

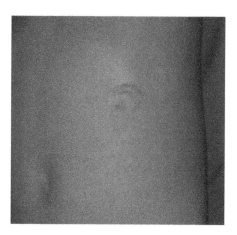

FIGURE 6.2.   Handlebar sign.

Reprinted from *Journal of Pediatric Surgery Case Reports*, vol 3, issue 5, R. Fernándeza, P. Bragagninia, N. Álvareza, R. Delgadoa, J. P. Garciab, R. Escartína, J. Graciaa, "Handlebar Injury in Children: Are We Ignoring the Signs?" Copyright 2015, with permission from Elsevier. https://doi.org/10.1016/j.epsc.2015.03.005

liver function tests, lipase, and urinalysis are indicated. Findings on laboratory exam suggestive of intra-abdominal injury in this context include elevated aspartate aminotransferase (AST) and alanine aminotransferase (ALT), hematuria, and an initial hematocrit less than 30%. Hemodynamic changes, including a low systolic blood pressure in the setting of blunt abdominal trauma supports a potential need for emergent surgical intervention, while hemodynamically stable patients may undergo CT imaging. Some institutions use the FAST exam to help guide decisions for further imaging. If the FAST exam is negative and CT imaging is not immediately obtained, we recommend serial clinical and laboratory exams for 24 hours, followed by CT imaging in the event of clinical deterioration.[13–15]

Abdominal Wall Contusions

Bruising on the abdomen in infants and children can also be a potential red-flag for nonaccidental trauma, particularly in the absence of a history of traumatic injury. While accidental bruising is a frequent occurrence in independently mobile infants/toddlers and school-aged children, the vast majority of these types of contusions occur over hard bony prominences including the shins, knees, forehead and occipital scalp. In contrast bruising in "soft" areas such as the cheeks, abdomen, back, chest, and buttocks is suggestive of abuse rather than accidental injury. The TEN4 is a clinical tool used to identify concerning bruising in children. This tool assesses for bruising over the torso, ears, or neck in children less than or equal to 4 years of age or any bruising in infants less than 4 months of age, and is predictive of abuse and a need for further investigation.[16]

Importantly, occult abusive abdominal trauma contributes to significant morbidity and mortality in pediatric patients. A large epidemiologic study in the United States found that more than 1 in 4 cases of abdominal trauma in children less than 1 year old were secondary to abuse.[17] Furthermore, abusive abdominal trauma is the second leading cause of death among physically abused children.[18] Blunt abusive abdominal trauma has been associated with injuries to every intra-abdominal organ, though most reports from the literature report highest rates of liver injury. Thus, the presence of abdominal bruising without an appropriate mechanism of injury should prompt further history and examination to investigate for nonaccidental trauma in addition to assessment of the abdomen to determine need for more urgent intervention.[18-21]

The presence of abdominal bruising should prompt clinicians to ask the family about the mechanism and timing of the injury. Additional history should attempt to elicit any concerning features for bleeding disorders such as a history of prolonged bleeding after procedures, epistaxis, or following minor injuries. Additionally, a family history focused on a history of excessive bleeding should also be obtained. Lastly, the clinician should conduct a complete psychosocial assessment to determine any potential risk factors for child maltreatment including young parental age, parental substance abuse, domestic violence, or financial stress.[18,21]

On physical examination of a child with abdominal bruising suspicious for nonaccidental trauma, it is important to document the size, color, location, and shape of the bruise. A thorough skin exam should be conducted to identify additional bruising or other patterned markings. Examination of the mouth and nares should attempt to identify nasal bleeding or intraoral injury, which can be highly suggestive of abuse in an infant. Musculoskeletal exam should attempt to identify any deformity, limited range of motion, or tenderness/swelling. As discussed earlier, in any child with abdominal bruising, the presence of abdominal tenderness or distension warrants further investigation. The clinician may consider a FAST exam, but ultimately a CT of the abdomen/pelvis should be obtained if there is concern for intra-abdominal injury. Additionally, laboratory evaluation to assess for solid organ injury as described previously is also recommended. In addition to consultation with the surgical team, consultation with a specialist in child abuse is also recommended. Physicians are mandated reporters of child abuse and therefore if suspicion of abuse persists, these concerns must be discussed with child protective services.[19–21]

CASE CONCLUSION

Back to our case! Intravenous access is obtained and the patient is given pain control with fentanyl and a bolus of lactated ringers. Her vital signs improved, however laboratory evaluation demonstrated elevated liver function tests and a mildly low hematocrit. She undergoes CT imaging which demonstrated thickening of the small bowel wall in multiple locations, and a small liver laceration and a fracture of L2/L3 with concern for three column disruption consistent with a Chance fracture. She underwent an exploratory laparotomy, which demonstrated a small bowel perforation and spinal stabilization. She remained neurologically intact postoperatively and was discharged on hospital day 10.

KEY POINTS TO REMEMBER

· Abdominal bruising in the pediatric patient is highly suggestive of significant blunt abdominal injury and is associated in a variety of contexts with both hollow viscus and solid organ injury.

· The seatbelt sign and handlebar mark warrants prompt imaging and laboratory examination.

· Abdominal bruising in pediatric patients without an overt history of trauma, or an inappropriate mechanism of trauma, is concerning for non-accidental injury.

Further Reading

1. Szadkowski MA, Bolte RG. Seatbelt syndrome in children. *Pediatr Emerg Care.* 2017;33(2):120–5. doi:10.1097/PEC.0000000000001027.
2. Lutz N, Nance ML, Kallan MJ, Arbogast KB, Durbin DR, Winston FK. Incidence and clinical significance of abdominal wall bruising in restrained children involved in motor vehicle crashes. *J Pediatr Surg.* 2004;39(6):972–5. doi:10.1016/j.jpedsurg.2004.02.029.
3. Borgialli DA, Ellison AM, Ehrlich P, et al. Association between the seat belt sign and intra-abdominal injuries in children with blunt torso trauma in motor vehicle collisions. Stevenson MD, ed. *Acad Emerg Med.* 2014;21(11):1240–8. doi:10.1111/acem.12506.
4. Holmes JF, Offerman SR, Chang CH, et al. Performance of helical computed tomography without oral contrast for the detection of gastrointestinal injuries. *Ann Emerg Med.* 2004;43(1):120–8. doi:10.1016/S0196-0644(03)00727-3.
5. Killeen KL, Shanmuganathan K, Poletti PA, Cooper C, Mirvis SE. Helical computed tomography of bowel and mesenteric injuries. *J Trauma.* 2001;51(1):26–36. doi:10.1097/00005373-200107000-00005.

6. Andras LM, Skaggs KF, Badkoobehi H, Choi PD, Skaggs DL. Chance fractures in the pediatric population are often misdiagnosed. *J Pediatr Orthop*. 2019;39(5):222–5. doi:10.1097/BPO.0000000000000925.

7. Arkader A, Warner WC, Tolo VT, Sponseller PD, Skaggs DL. Pediatric Chance fractures: a multicenter perspective. *J Pediatr Orthop*. 2011;31(7):741–4. doi:10.1097/BPO.0b013e31822f1b0b.

8. Achildi O, Betz RR, Grewal H. Lapbelt injuries and the seatbelt syndrome in pediatric spinal cord injury. *J Spinal Cord Med*. 2007;30(Suppl 1):S21–4. doi:10.1080/10790268.2007.11753964.

9. Winston FK, Shaw KN, Kreshak AA, Schwarz DF, Gallagher PR, Cnaan A. Hidden spears: handlebars as injury hazards to children. *Pediatrics*. 1998;102(3 Pt 1):596–601. doi:10.1542/peds.102.3.596.

10. Nadler EP, Potoka DA, Shultz BL, Morrison KE, Ford HR, Gaines BA. The high morbidity associated with handlebar injuries in children. *J Trauma*. 2005;58(6):1171–4. doi:10.1097/01.TA.0000170107.21534.7A.

11. Nance ML, Keller MS, Stafford PW. Predicting hollow visceral injury in the pediatric blunt trauma patient with solid visceral injury. *J Pediatr Surg*. 2000;35(9):1300–1303. doi:10.1053/jpsu.2000.9301.

12. Rathore A, Simpson BJ, Diefenbach KA. Traumatic abdominal wall hernias: an emerging trend in handlebar injuries. *J Pediatr Surg*. 2012;47(7):1410–3. doi:10.1016/j.jpedsurg.2012.02.003.

13. Klimek PM, Lutz T, Stranzinger E, Zachariou Z, Kessler U, Berger S. Handlebar injuries in children. *Pediatr Surg Int*. 2012;29(3):269–73. doi:10.1007/s00383-012-3227-y.

14. Notrica DM. Pediatric blunt abdominal trauma. *Curr Opin Crit Care*. 2015;21(6):531–7. doi:10.1097/MCC.0000000000000249.

15. Fernández R, Bragagnini P, Álvarez N, et al. Handlebar injury in children: are we ignoring the signs? *J Pediatr Surg Case Rep*. 2015;3(5):215–8. doi:10.1016/j.epsc.2015.03.005.

16. Pierce MC, Kaczor K, Aldridge S, O'Flynn J, Lorenz DJ. Bruising characteristics discriminating physical child abuse from accidental trauma. *Pediatrics*. 2010;125(1):67–74. doi:10.1542/peds.2008-3632.

17. Lane WG, Dubowitz H, Langenberg P, Dischinger P. Epidemiology of abusive abdominal trauma hospitalizations in United States children. *Child Abuse and Neglect*. 2012;36(2):142–8. doi:10.1016/j.chiabu.2011.09.010.

18. Glick JC, Lorand MA, Bilka KR. Physical abuse of children. *Pediatr Rev*. 2016;37(4):146–56–quiz157. doi:10.1542/pir.2015-0012.

19. Paul AR, Adamo MA. Non-accidental trauma in pediatric patients: a review of epidemiology, pathophysiology, diagnosis and treatment. *Transl Pediatr*. 2014;3(3):195–207. doi:10.3978/j.issn.2224-4336.2014.06.01.

20. Barnes PM, Norton CM, Dunstan FD, Kemp AM, Yates DW, Sibert JR. Abdominal injury due to child abuse. *Lancet*. 2005;366(9481):234–5. doi:10.1016/S0140-6736(05)66913-9.
21. Christian CW, Committee on Child Abuse and Neglect, American Academy of Pediatrics. The evaluation of suspected child physical abuse. *Pediatrics*. 2015;135(5):e1337–54. doi:10.1542/peds.2015-0356.

7 My Belly Hurts—And I Got Hit by the Hulk

Seth Linakis

A healthy 15-year-old boy presents to the emergency department with abdominal pain and nausea. He reports having been kneed in the left side of his abdomen by a larger athlete during a soccer game about three hours prior to presentation. Although initially minor, his pain has been progressively worsening. Ambulation leads to increased abdominal discomfort. Ibuprofen en route did not alleviate his pain. He has no chronic medical conditions, does not take any medications regularly, and has no known allergies. He is triaged as a Level 2 trauma. His primary survey has the following findings: heart rate 125 bpm, respirations 20 bpm, pulse oximetry 100% on room air, blood pressure 106/70. He is pale and ill appearing. His secondary survey was significant for a diffusely tender but soft abdomen with no distension, no external markings, and no peritoneal signs. His rectal exam is negative for blood and there is no gross hematuria. A FAST scan does not demonstrate any free fluid.

What do you do now?

HIGH-GRADE LIVER LACERATION

Diagnosis

Abdominal trauma is a significant cause of morbidity and mortality in children, and multiple features of this patient's presentation should cause concern. First and foremost, although tachycardia could be present in this patient for many reasons, in the context of his history and other clinical findings it is appropriate to assume normotensive shock. This is particularly true in an athlete whose baseline heart rate is likely significantly lower than average. Second, the relatively rapid progression of symptoms also suggests more serious intra-abdominal pathology. Third, although ultrasound FAST scans are becoming more prevalent, the limitations of the study must be taken into account—a negative FAST does not exclude intra-abdominal bleeding.

The differential diagnosis for a pediatric patient presenting with diffuse pain after abdominal trauma is relatively broad. In addition to solid organ lacerations (liver, spleen, pancreas, kidneys), hollow viscus injuries such as perforation or contusion should be considered. The bladder may also be injured, which will generally result in the presence of hematuria. Although rare, a patient with respiratory distress after abdominal injury may have suffered a diaphragmatic rupture. An abdominal wall contusion would be unlikely to produce the symptoms seen in this patient and in any case should be a diagnosis of exclusion.

The initial trauma primary and secondary surveys are critical to narrow the differential and direct management. As with any trauma, the patient's airway, breathing, and circulation claim top priority. However, there are several findings on the secondary survey that may be useful. Abdominal ecchymoses in the setting of trauma can be highly suggestive of hemorrhage, especially in patients brought from the scene of motor vehicle crashes ("seatbelt sign"). Additionally, although often deferred (or omitted entirely), a digital rectal exam, which has been shown to have very low sensitivity as a screening test is however very helpful if abnormal and can provide crucial data: frank blood on the exam suggests the presence of hollow viscus injury. This is particularly important given that the sensitivity of abdominal CT for hollow viscus injury is only around 80%. Undetected hollow viscus injury can have potentially devastating consequences with significant morbidity (e.g., peritonitis). As a result, early detection may be life-saving for the patient. Careful evaluation of the pelvis is also warranted, as bedside imaging such as FAST will not identify pelvic hemorrhage. Finally, left shoulder pain after abdominal trauma (known as the Kehr sign) may suggest subphrenic blood from a splenic laceration.

Along with the trauma survey and appropriate stabilization, multiple other studies and interventions should be performed on a pediatric patient presenting with potentially severe blunt abdominal trauma. Gastric decompression with an orogastric tube (or nasogastric tube in the absence of facial trauma) serves multiple functions. It can alleviate abdominal distension, improving the quality of serial exams and preventing thoracic compression with the attendant respiratory compromise, and it empties the stomach of fluid (blood or otherwise) which both removes a potential source of gastroenteric irritation and minimizes the risk of aspiration. Some laboratory testing may be useful and is often necessary. In order to expedite future transfusions, particularly if the patient undergoes a surgical procedure, send a sample as early as possible for type and screen or cross-match. A complete blood count or hemoglobin + hematocrit (H&H) is typically sent on presentation; however, the initial result must be treated cautiously (or used as a baseline depending on timing) as it may take up to 4 hours for the test to reflect the true values accurately in the setting of acute blood loss. The utility of transaminases has been hotly debated in the literature. Many cutoffs have been proposed to delineate risk for serious hepatic injury, but there is no real consensus. As a result, there are no unified recommendations regarding interpretation of transaminase levels, although they are still recommended for a patient with blunt abdominal trauma. Grossly bloody urine suggests kidney or bladder injury and should be obtained if there is no evidence of urethral injury. A lipase level is useful to evaluate for pancreatic injury, and many sources suggest that an amylase may also be helpful in the setting of trauma. In a stable patient, additional testing including bedside chest and pelvis films may be considered as a part of the secondary survey. One other pathology that must be considered, especially in patients brought in from motor vehicle collisions, is a Chance fracture. This is a flexion-distraction injury of the lumbar spine that most often results from wearing a lap belt incorrectly. While neurologic sequelae are uncommon, up to half of patients with Chance fractures have associated intra-abdominal injuries, with a high frequency of hollow viscus pathology.

Our patient's abdominal exam continued to worsen in the emergency department, so a FAST scan was repeated and demonstrated free fluid inside the liver capsule (Figure 7.1). After initial stabilization with crystalloid fluids and surgical consultation, a CT scan of the abdomen and pelvis with IV contrast was obtained. This demonstrated a stellate liver laceration characterized as grade IV (parenchymal involvement of 25%–75% of a hepatic lobe or evidence of intraparenchymal bleeding with extension into the peritoneum) as well as a grade I splenic laceration (capsular tear with < 1 cm parenchymal depth) and a grade I injury of the superior pole of the right kidney (subcapsular hematoma, nonexpanding, no parenchymal laceration). There was no evidence of free air or hollow viscus injury.

While abdominal trauma in children is relatively common, it is less common to see such injuries in the context of sports participation. Those that do occur are more common in boys than in girls (approximately 4:1) and are more likely to happen in children over 12 years old. As with most

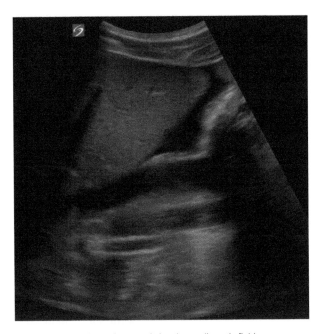

FIGURE 7.1. Right upper quadrant ultrasound showing perihepatic fluid.

pathologies, the key to timely diagnosis is a focused, accurate history, and physical exam.

The value of imaging in these patients is a matter of some debate. Older management guidelines were based primarily on the grade of injury as determined by CT scan (Table 7.1). Decisions regarding ICU admission and surgical intervention relied on what the imaging showed. More recently, however, this approach has been largely replaced by a more patient-centered model in which management decisions rely primarily on hemodynamic status and response to therapy, and imaging is used more to assist in the planning of an invasive intervention (e.g., embolization or laparotomy). The approach recommended by the Pediatric Trauma Society (PTS), initially developed by the Arizona-Texas-Oklahoma-Memphis-Arkansas Consortium (ATOMAC), includes imaging as part of the process, but all decision points are made on the basis of clinical status and hemoglobin/hematocrit trend. Ultimately, nonoperative management has become the standard of care in the vast majority of these injuries.

Based on the ATOMAC guidelines, our patient was initially admitted to the PICU for serial exams and H&H monitoring. Despite his grade IV liver laceration, his H&H and hemodynamic status remained stable after admission and he was transferred to the floor on hospital day 1. He did not

TABLE 7.1. **CT Grading of Liver Lacerations**

Grade	Description
I	Laceration of hepatic parenchyma < 1 cm deep; no length criteria
II	Laceration of hepatic parenchyma 1–3 cm deep; must also be ≤10 cm long
III	Laceration of hepatic parenchyma >3 cm deep OR evidence of active intraparenchymal bleeding WITHOUT extension into the peritoneum
IV	Disruption of 25%–75% of a hepatic lobe OR evidence of active intraparenchymal bleeding WITH extension into the peritoneum
V	Disruption of >75% of a hepatic lobe OR juxtahepatic venous injury

*Modified from: Kozar RA, Crandall M, Shanmuganathan K, et al. Organ injury scaling 2018 update: spleen, liver, and kidney. *J Trauma Acute Care Surg.* 2018;85:1119.

receive any blood products and did not undergo any embolization or surgical procedures. He was ultimately discharged on hospital day 3 without any complications. The surgery team recommended 6 weeks of activity restriction, which he completed without complication and was cleared for full return to sports. It is important to note that discharge recommendations for abdominal solid organ injuries are not standardized. Generally, patients are held out of athletics and similarly strenuous activities until cleared by a pediatric surgeon. While 6 weeks is a relatively common time frame, it is far from universal.

In summary, blunt abdominal injuries in pediatric patients occur under a variety of circumstances. They can be life-threatening, so a high clinical index of suspicion is warranted with a concerning history and/or progressive exam. Evaluation and stabilization should be performed rapidly, and ongoing management determined with a pediatric surgeon based on the patient's hemodynamic status. Overall, with appropriate management, children who suffer solid abdominal organ lacerations or related injuries do exceedingly well, with less than 5% undergoing surgical intervention.

KEY POINTS TO REMEMBER

· The spleen is the most common abdominal solid organ lacerated, followed by the liver.
· Patients with abdominal solid organ injuries may not have significant external findings (e.g. ecchymosis), so a high degree of clinical suspicion is important in making the diagnosis early.
· A negative FAST scan does not rule out solid organ injury or intra-abdominal bleeding.
· While an abdominal CT is potentially useful for defining solid organ injuries, particularly prior to surgical intervention, appropriate management is based on hemodynamic status rather than the radiographic grade of the injury.
· The vast majority (~95%) of pediatric patients with blunt liver or spleen trauma recover fully with nonoperative management.
· Return to play guidelines are not standardized; activity limitations should be monitored by a pediatric surgeon.

Further Reading

Fremgen HE, Bratton SL, Metzger RR, Barnhart DC. Pediatric liver lacerations and intensive care: evaluation of ICU triage strategies. *Pediatr Crit Care Med*. 2014;15(4):e183–91.

Holmes JF, Kelley KM, Wootton-Gorges SL, et al. Organ injury scaling 2018 update: spleen, liver, and kidney. *J Trauma Acute Care Surg*. 2018;85:1119.

Holmes JF, Lillis K, Monroe D, Borgialli D, Kerrey BT, et al. Identifying children at very low risk of clinically important blunt abdominal trauma. *Ann Emerg Med*. 2013;62:107–16.

Kopelman TR, Jamshidi R, Pieri PG, et al. Computed tomographic imaging in the pediatric patient with a seatbelt sign: still not good enough. *J Pediatr Surg*. 2018;53(2):357–61.

Kupperman N. Effect of abdominal ultrasound on clinical care, outcomes, and resource use among children with blunt torso trauma. *JAMA*. 2017;317(22):2290–6.

McVay MR, Kokoska ER, Jackson RJ, Smith SD. Throwing out the "grade" book: management of isolated spleen and liver injury based on hemodynamic status. *J Pediatr Surg*. 2008;43:1072–6.

Notrica DM, Eubanks JW III, Tuggle DW, et al. Nonoperative management of blunt liver and spleen injury in children: evaluation of the ATOMAC guideline using GRADE. *J Trauma Acute Care Surg*. 2015;79:683–93.

Saladino RA, Lund DP. Abdominal trauma. In: Shaw KN, Bachur RG, eds. *Fleisher and Ludwig's Textbook of Pediatric Emergency Medicine*. 7th ed. Philadelphia, PA: Wolters Kluwer; 2016:1115–25.

Scaife ER, Rollins MD, Barnhart DC, et al. The role of focused abdominal sonography for trauma (FAST) in pediatric trauma evaluation. *J Pediatr Surg*. 2013;48:1377–83.

Visenio MR, Buesing KL, Moffatt K. Solid organ laceration in an adolescent soccer player: a case report. *Med Sci Sports Exerc*. 2017;49(10):1975–9.

8 The Rocking Pelvis

Hoi See Tsao and Robyn Wing

A 14-year-old female presents to the emergency
department after being struck by a motor vehicle
while crossing the road. Emergency medical services
report that there was intrusion into the vehicle and
that she was nonambulatory at the scene. She is alert
and responsive and when questioned, she complains
of severe pain in her back and both hips that is worse
with any movement. She was feeling well prior to
the accident, with no medical problems and takes
no home medications. Her heart rate is 110 beats
per minute and her blood pressure is 90/60 mmHg.
Examination is notable for tenderness to palpation
over the sacrum and bilateral iliac crests. Downward
and medial pressure over the pelvic iliac wings
reveals laxity. Genitourinary exam reveals blood at
the vaginal introitus.

What do you do now?

PELVIC TRAUMA

Pediatric pelvic fractures are rare and identified in 5% of children admitted to level 1 trauma centers after blunt trauma. The 5% overall mortality rate for pediatric pelvic fractures is usually due to fracture-induced fatal exsanguination which is lower than in adults, which is estimated to be 17%.[1,2] It is important to correctly identify and manage these injuries due to the potential for life-threatening hemorrhage from the presacral and lumbar venous plexuses with an unstable pelvic fracture and to ensure that pelvic fractures are followed closely to maximize normal pelvic growth and healing and avoid limb-length discrepancies and nerve deficits.[1,3]

The pelvic and genitourinary physical examinations are highly sensitive for significant pelvic fractures in trauma patients with Glasgow Coma Scale (GCS) scores of 14 or 15 and findings guide further workup and management.[4] Physical examination should include inspection for external bleeding, ecchymosis (perineal, scrotal, or flank), blood at the penile meatus and vaginal introitus, and the positioning of the lower extremities and iliac crests. This should be followed by palpation of bony landmarks, range of motion testing (assuming no deformity or pain) and assessment for neurovascular integrity. The rectum and vagina should be examined to assess for open fractures.[5] Pelvic stability is evaluated by applying gentle downward and medial pressure on the pelvis while the patient is lying supine. Once a pelvic injury is suspected, repeated pelvic compressions should be avoided to prevent fracture displacement, exacerbation of previous injuries and further hemorrhage.[5,6]

There are three main mechanisms of injuries for pelvic fractures: lateral compression, anterior–posterior compression, and vertical shear.[6] In adults, 60%–70% of pelvic fractures are due to lateral compression, 15%–20% are due to anterior–posterior compression and 5%–15% are due to vertical shear.[6] Children have more pliable bones and stronger ligaments than adults, making isolated pelvic ring fractures and avulsion fractures of the pelvis more common in children.[5] The term "open-book pelvic fracture" is commonly used to describe pelvic ring disruptions that result in anterior ring widening and a posterior pelvic fracture or ligamentous injury.[5] An open-book fracture is most typically associated with an anterior–posterior compression mechanism of injury[6] but can occur with any mechanism of injury.[5]

Initial diagnostic testing includes a bedside focused assessment with sonography in trauma (FAST) examination due to its availability and high specificity.[7,8] However, further evaluation to elucidate specific injuries with plain radiography or computed tomography (CT) is needed if the FAST scan is negative and clinical suspicion for pelvic injury remains. Although a portable plain anterior–posterior radiograph has low sensitivity, it may be a valuable adjunct in unstable patients to assess for significantly displaced fractures that may be causing hemorrhage, as in the case of this patient (Figure 8.1).[9–12] In addition, she should have a CT scan of the pelvis, which is the gold standard for diagnosing pelvic injuries due to its high sensitivity.[13]

The American College of Surgeons previously recommended that any patient with blunt trauma should have a routine pelvic radiograph.[14] However, this can lead to unnecessary costs, delays in management, and radiation exposure in the pediatric blunt trauma population.[14] Studies have shown that pelvic radiographs can be eliminated with high negative predictive value in

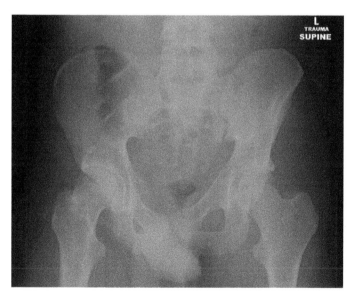

FIGURE 8.1. X-ray showing multiple pelvic fractures including left sacroiliac fracture dislocation and left acetabulum anterior column fracture. Radiologic interpretation and image courtesy of Dr. Thaddeus Herliczek.

the trauma workup of hemodynamically stable pediatric patients with GCS scores of 14 or 15 who do not have lower extremity injuries (hip held in rotation at presentation, hip deformity or pain), have a normal pelvic physical examination (no pelvic tenderness, laceration, ecchymosis, abrasion), no back pain, no abdominal pain or tenderness, negative urinalysis for blood, and no high-risk mechanism of injury (unrestrained motor vehicle collision, motor vehicle collision with ejection, motor vehicle rollover, automobile vs. pedestrian or automobile vs. bicycle).[14–17]

Initial management should focus on stabilization of the airway, breathing, and circulation in the primary survey, as recommended by the Advanced Trauma Life Support (ATLS) guidelines. This patient's tachycardia and borderline blood pressure in the setting of a potential pelvic fracture are highly suggestive of hemorrhagic shock. If a significant pelvic injury is suspected, particularly in the setting of hemodynamic instability, both fluid resuscitation and hemorrhage control are of utmost importance.[6] Fluid resuscitation can be achieved with intravenous fluids and blood transfusions. As pelvic fractures are associated with a high incidence of internal injuries and bleeding, consideration should be given to initiation of a massive transfusion protocol early in the trauma evaluation.[5] A portable plain anterior–posterior radiograph of the pelvis has low sensitivity of 50% to 80% for pediatric pelvic fractures but should be used in this tachycardic and hypotensive patient to assess for significantly displaced fractures that may be causing hemorrhage.[9–12] Hemorrhage control is achieved through mechanical stabilization of the pelvis with the goal of reducing pelvic volume. There are several ways to do this, including taping the lower extremities in internal rotation and tightly wrapping a sheet, pelvic binder, or other device at the level of the greater trochanters of the femur (not the level of the pelvic iliac crests).[5,6] These maneuvers are temporizing measures, and specialist consultation needs to be obtained early in the evaluation for definitive management of pelvic injuries with trauma surgery, orthopedic surgery, and interventional radiology if available. Often, ongoing hemorrhage in the setting of pelvic fractures is best managed by angiographic embolization.[6]

Pelvic fractures are frequently associated with urethral injuries, which have a high complication rate.[6,18] If physical examination reveals blood at the urethral meatus, a high-riding prostate, or gross hematuria, a retrograde urethrogram should be performed prior to Foley catheter placement to assess for urethral injury. In females, a retrograde urethrogram should also be performed if there is blood at the vaginal introitus, as in this case, given that urethral injuries are frequently associated with laceration of the vaginal wall in the setting of pelvic fractures.[19] Urethral injuries are categorized into those above (posterior) or below (anterior) the urogenital diaphragm. Patients with multisystem injuries and pelvic fractures typically have posterior urethral injuries while anterior urethral injuries are more likely to be isolated or from straddle injuries.[6] While there is a lower incidence of genitourinary injury in pediatric patients with pelvic fractures, they are frequently overlooked in children in the emergency department and potentially worsened with placement of a urinary catheter.[19] They therefore require a high index of suspicion and any concerning findings on the genitourinary examination, or if the patient has gross hematuria or inability to void, should prompt consideration for a retrograde urethrogram.[19,20]

High-energy mechanisms of injury, such as in this case that resulted in significant pelvic trauma, may in addition, inflict other internal injuries including intraabdominal injuries. In adults, the severity of pelvic fractures is often associated with the severity of concurrent splenic and hepatic injuries and warrants close monitoring and management.[21] The same correlation has not been found in children but should still necessitate a detailed abdominal physical examination in the setting of severe trauma to determine the need for further abdominal workup or imaging.[21] Finally, while uncommon, in both adults and children, pelvic injuries are associated with rectal injury.[21] If unnoticed, rectal injuries can lead to serious infection including sepsis and death,[22] highlighting the importance of a thorough physical examination.

Treatment of pelvic fractures depends on the age of the patient, fracture type, pelvic ring stability, concomitant injuries, and hemodynamic stability. The majority of pediatric pelvic fractures are treated nonsurgically with a small number needing reduction and fixation.[3] While pelvic injuries are rare, the implications are great including the potential for hemorrhage, long-term effects on development and growth if unrecognized, and association with other injuries due to the high-energy mechanism of the trauma. Appropriate workup and management must therefore be individualized for each patient based on a thorough physical exam with a high index of suspicion for concomitant injuries.

· Pediatric pelvic injuries indicate a high-energy mechanism and warrant an evaluation for concomitant abdominal and genitourinary injuries.
· Use plain radiography and CT to evaluate for pelvic injuries.
· Volume resuscitation and hemorrhage control can be achieved in the setting of an unstable pelvis with intravenous fluids and blood products and by applying a sheet or pelvic binder around the pelvis to reduce pelvic volume.
· Perform a retrograde urethrogram if there is blood at the vaginal introitus, blood at the urethral meatus, a high-riding prostate, gross hematuria, or inability to void.
· Initiation of massive transfusion protocols and consultation to trauma surgery, orthopedic surgery, and interventional radiology should be considered when a significant pelvic injury is suspected.

Further Reading
1. DeFrancesco CJ, Sankar WN. Traumatic pelvic fractures in children and adolescents. *Semin Pediatr Surg.* 2017;26(1):27–35. doi: 10.1053/j.sempedsurg.2017.01.006[published Online First: Epub Date]|.
2. Ismail N, Bellemare JF, Mollitt DL, DiScala C, Koeppel B, Tepas JJ 3rd. Death from pelvic fracture: children are different. *J Pediatr Surg.* 1996;31(1):82–85.
3. Holden CP, Holman J, Herman MJ. Pediatric pelvic fractures. *J Am Acad Orthop Surg.* 2007;15(3):172–7.
4. Gonzalez RP, Fried PQ, Bukhalo M. The utility of clinical examination in screening for pelvic fractures in blunt trauma. *J Am Coll Surg.* 2002;194(2):121–5.
5. Fiechtl J. Pelvic trauma: Initial evaluation and management. In: J Grayzel, ed. UpToDate, 2018. Waltham, MA: UpToDate Inc. https://www.uptodate.com/contents/pelvic-trauma-initial-evaluation-and-management?search=pelvic%20trauma&source=search_result&selectedTitle=1~150&usage_type=default&display_rank=1 (Accessed on December 1, 2018).
6. ATLS Subcommittee; American College of Surgeons' Committee on Trauma, International ATLS Working Group. Advanced trauma life support (ATLS®): the ninth edition. *J Trauma Acute Care Surg.* 2013;74(5):1363–6. doi: 10.1097/TA.0b013e31828b82f5[published Online First: Epub Date]|.

7. Friese RS, Malekzadeh S, Shafi S, Gentilello LM, Starr A. Abdominal ultrasound is an unreliable modality for the detection of hemoperitoneum in patients with pelvic fracture. *J Trauma*. 2007;63(1):97–102. doi: 10.1097/TA.0b013e31805f6ffb[published Online First: Epub Date]|.

8. Tayal VS, Nielsen A, Jones AE, Thomason MH, Kellam J, Norton HJ. Accuracy of trauma ultrasound in major pelvic injury. *J Trauma*. 2006;61(6):1453–7. doi: 10.1097/01.ta.0000197434.58433.88[published Online First: Epub Date]|.

9. Kessel B, Sevi R, Jeroukhimov I, et al. Is routine portable pelvic X-ray in stable multiple trauma patients always justified in a high technology era? *Injury*. 2007;38(5):559–63. doi: 10.1016/j.injury.2006.12.020[published Online First: Epub Date]|.

10. Obaid AK, Barleben A, Porral D, Lush S, Cinat M. Utility of plain film pelvic radiographs in blunt trauma patients in the emergency department. *Am Surg*. 2006;72(10):951–4.

11. Guillamondegui OD, Mahboubi S, Stafford PW, Nance ML. The utility of the pelvic radiograph in the assessment of pediatric pelvic fractures. *J Trauma*. 2003;55(2):236–9; discussion 39–40. doi: 10.1097/01.TA.0000079250.80811.D1[published Online First: Epub Date]|.

12. Kwok MY, Yen K, Atabaki S, et al. Sensitivity of plain pelvis radiography in children with blunt torso trauma. *Ann Emerg Med*. 2015;65(1):63–71. doi: 10.1016/j.annemergmed.2014.06.017[published Online First: Epub Date]|.

13. Vela JH, Wertz CI, Onstott KL, Wertz JR. Trauma imaging: a literature review. *Radiol Technol*. 2017;88(3):263–76.

14. Wong AT, Brady KB, Caldwell AM, Graber NM, Rubin DH, Listman DA. Low-risk criteria for pelvic radiography in pediatric blunt trauma patients. *Pediatr Emerg Care*. 2011;27(2):92–96. doi: 10.1097/PEC.0b013e3182094355[published Online First: Epub Date]|.

15. Haasz M, Simone LA, Wales PW, et al. Which pediatric blunt trauma patients do not require pelvic imaging? *J Trauma Acute Care Surg*. 2015;79(5):828–32. doi: 10.1097/TA.0000000000000848[published Online First: Epub Date]|.

16. Lagisetty J, Slovis T, Thomas R, Knazik S, Stankovic C. Are routine pelvic radiographs in major pediatric blunt trauma necessary? *Pediatr Radiol*. 2012;42(7):853–8. doi: 10.1007/s00247-011-2341-7[published Online First: Epub Date]|.

17. Ramirez DW, Schuette JJ, Knight V, Johnson E, Denise J, Walker AR. Necessity of routine pelvic radiograph in the pediatric blunt trauma patient. *Clin Pediatr (Phila)*. 2008;47(9):935–40. doi: 10.1177/0009922808320598[published Online First: Epub Date]|.

18. Hagedorn JC, Voelzke BB. Pelvic-fracture urethral injury in children. *Arab J Urol*. 2015;13(1):37–42. doi: 10.1016/j.aju.2014.11.007[published Online First: Epub Date]|.

19. Meltzer JA, Reddy SH, Blumfield E, Alvayay C, Blumberg SM. Pelvic fracture urethral injuries in children: a case report and appraisal of their emergency management. *Pediatr Emerg Care*. 2016;32(9):627–9. doi: 10.1097/PEC.0000000000000534[published Online First: Epub Date]|.

20. Tarman GJ, Kaplan GW, Lerman SL, McAleer IM, Losasso BE. Lower genitourinary injury and pelvic fractures in pediatric patients. *Urology*. 2002;59(1):123–6; discussion 26.

21. Swaid F, Peleg K, Alfici R, et al. A comparison study of pelvic fractures and associated abdominal injuries between pediatric and adult blunt trauma patients. *J Pediatr Surg*. 2017;52(3):386–9. doi: 10.1016/j.jpedsurg.2016.09.055[published Online First: Epub Date]|.

22. Song W, Zhou D, Xu W, et al. Factors of pelvic infection and death in patients with open pelvic fractures and rectal injuries. *Surg Infect (Larchmt)*. 2017;18(6):711–5. doi: 10.1089/sur.2017.083[published Online First: Epub Date]|.

9 Is FAST Too FAST?

Laurie Malia and Joni E. Rabiner

A 10-year-old previously healthy male is brought in by emergency medical services (EMS) to the emergency department (ED) after being struck by a car. EMS reports that he ran into the street to retrieve a ball and was struck in his left flank by a sedan traveling about 25 mph. Witnesses reported that he flew in the air 5 feet and landed on his back. There was no loss of consciousness. On arrival to the ED, he is awake and alert but complaining of diffuse abdominal pain. His vital signs are: temperature 37°C, heart rate 102 bpm, respiratory rate 22 breaths per minute, blood pressure 125/78, and pulse oximetry 98% on room air. On primary survey, his airway is patent, trachea is midline, lungs are clear bilaterally, and he has warm upper and lower extremities bilaterally with 2+ radial and pedal pulses. On secondary survey, notable findings include diffuse abdominal tenderness with guarding most severe in the left upper quadrant. He is neurovascularly intact.

What do you do now?

DISCUSSION

In this previously healthy boy struck by a motor vehicle sustaining blunt abdominal trauma, the major concern is for intra-abdominal injury, including hematoma or laceration of the liver, spleen, pancreas, or intestines. Retroperitoneal injury, including injury to the kidneys, and superficial musculoskeletal or soft tissue abdominal injury, are also on the differential diagnosis. Blunt abdominal trauma occurs in 10%–15% of children who present with traumatic injuries, with the spleen being the most commonly injured organ.[1,2] This patient sustained blunt trauma and has abdominal pain and guarding, particularly in the left upper quadrant, and therefore his presentation is most concerning for splenic injury with intra-peritoneal bleeding. The patient is tachycardic, but has a normal blood pressure.

As intravenous access is obtained, determine what laboratory studies and imaging tests are needed. Standard trauma evaluation laboratory tests are sent. The trauma team is present and is debating awaiting laboratory results versus immediately obtaining a CT scan of the abdomen. The value of a point-of-care focused assessment with sonography for trauma (FAST) examination should be determined, based on the clinical status of the patient and resources available at the institution.

The FAST examination provides quick, reliable information on bleeding into the peritoneal, pericardial, and pleural spaces in the setting of trauma. The FAST is noninvasive and repeatable and does not involve ionizing radiation or time delays, which makes it an ideal first-line test in pediatric trauma patients. It is part of the Advanced Trauma Life Support (ATLS) protocol, and it can be performed immediately after the primary survey simultaneously with other resuscitative measures as needed. The FAST has been shown to detect as little as 250 mL of free fluid and is more accurate in ruling in rather than ruling out intra-abdominal injury.[3] While the FAST exam is most useful for detection of clinically significant intra-abdominal injury requiring operative intervention, it is important to recognize that the FAST is not reliable for detecting solid organ, retroperitoneal, or hollow viscous (bowel) injuries. The extended FAST, or eFAST, adds evaluation of the lungs for hemothorax or pneumothorax to the bedside ultrasound exam.

The FAST exam evaluates four locations of the abdomen for free fluid: right upper quadrant, left upper quadrant, pelvis, and subxiphoid. The right upper quadrant view assesses Morison's pouch or the hepatorenal recess, which is the most dependent area of the upper abdomen, for free fluid. The left upper quadrant view evaluates the splenorenal recess for free fluid, and the area between the diaphragm and spleen needs to be assessed for free fluid as well. In both the right and left upper quadrant views, it is important to visualize the inferior pole of the kidney, as this may be the first site of small fluid accumulation. In addition, in the right and left upper quadrant views, the probe may be moved cephalad or fanned above the diaphragm to assess the costophrenic angles for free fluid, or hemothorax, as part of the eFAST exam. The suprapubic view evaluates the rectovesicular pouch in males or the pouch of Douglas between the uterus and rectum in females for free fluid—these have been found to be the most common sites of fluid accumulation in children.[4] The subxiphoid pericardial view evaluates for free fluid in the pericardial space. For the eFAST exam, the anterior lungs may be assessed for pneumothorax as well.

How accurate is the FAST exam for detection of free fluid, and does it have an effect on clinical outcomes? In a 2018 Cochrane Database Systematic Review of FAST in adults and children with blunt abdominal trauma including 34 studies with 8,635 patients, the overall sensitivity was 74% and specificity was 96%.[5] When looking at the 10 studies with 1,384 pediatric patients, the sensitivity was 63% and specificity was 91%.[5] A randomized controlled trial of FAST versus standard trauma care in adults showed that those that had a FAST exam performed had decreased time to operative care, decreased complications, decreased CT utilization, decreased hospital length of stay, and decreased costs.[6] However, a randomized controlled trial of hemodynamically stable children with blunt abdominal trauma that looked at FAST performed by ED physicians versus no FAST found that rates of CT use, time to CT scan, missed intra-abdominal injuries, ED length of stay, and cost were not statistically different between the two groups.[7] In addition, it has been shown that serial FAST exams can significantly increase the sensitivity of the FAST exam.[8]

What is the utility of the FAST exam in blunt abdominal trauma? Ultimately, FAST can be a useful tool, with higher sensitivities and specificities in adult studies than in pediatric studies. The FAST can be most helpful in hemodynamically unstable patients with abdominal free fluid identified on FAST and can facilitate the decision to immediately take the patient to the operating room. A negative FAST must be interpreted carefully within the clinical context, and history including mechanism of injury, physical examination, and laboratory findings can help to direct further evaluation and management. In a low-risk patient with a negative FAST exam, it may be possible to forgo additional imaging. However, when there remains high suspicion for intra-abdominal injury, despite a negative FAST exam, further diagnostic imaging should be pursued, as a negative FAST does not exclude intra-abdominal injuries.

As for our patient, a FAST exam is performed by the emergency medicine physician and identifies small free fluid in the splenorenal space (Figure 9.1). Since he has significant left upper quadrant pain with guarding and a FAST exam positive for free fluid but is hemodynamically stable, the decision is made to obtain an abdominal CT scan, which shows a grade 3 splenic laceration. His laboratory tests show a hemoglobin of 7.4 g/dL, hematocrit of 28%, and normal liver function tests and coagulation studies. His urinalysis is negative for blood. The patient is admitted to the hospital for serial abdominal exams and monitoring of his hemoglobin/hematocrit. He is discharged 5 days later with a stable hemoglobin and hematocrit.

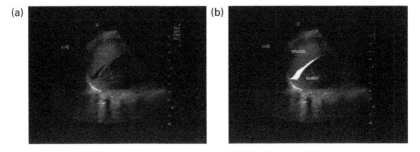

FIGURE 9.1. Left upper quadrant FAST view showing free fluid in the splenorenal space (a) and with spleen, kidney, and free fluid labeled (b). Image courtesy of Dr. Anju Wagh.

· Blunt abdominal trauma is common in pediatric patients.

· The FAST examination has been shown to be highly specific in identifying children with hemoperitoneum; however, it is less accurate for ruling out hemoperitoneum and intra-abdominal injury.

· For a patient with blunt abdominal trauma with a positive FAST exam, those that are hemodynamically unstable should be taken directly to the operating room while those that are hemodynamically stable may be assessed with further abdominal imaging.

· For a patient with blunt abdominal trauma and a negative FAST exam, further management is directed by the clinical suspicion for clinically significant intra-abdominal injury based on the mechanism of injury, physical examination findings, laboratory findings, and local trauma protocols or trauma team input.

· A negative FAST exam in a patient at low risk for intra-abdominal injury may decrease CT scan rates.

Further Reading

1. Gaines BA. Intra-abdominal solid organ injury in children: diagnosis and treatment. *J Trauma.* 2009;67(2 Suppl):S135.

2. Wilson RH, Moorehead RJ. Management of splenic trauma. *Injury.* 1992;23(1):5.

3. Branney SW, Wolfe RE, Moore EE, et al. Quantitative sensitivity of ultrasound in detecting intraperitoneal fluid. *J Trauma.* 1995;39(2):375–80.

4. Nance ML, Mahboubi S, Wickstrom M, et al. Pattern of abdominal free fluid following isolated blunt spleen or liver injury in the pediatric patient. *J Trauma.* 2002;52(1):85–7.

5. Stengel D, Leisterer J, Ferrada P, et al. Point-of-care ultrasonography for diagnosing thoracoabdominal injuries in patients with blunt trauma. *Cochrane Database of Syst Rev.* 2018; 12. doi: 10.1002/14651858.CD012669.pub2.

6. Melniker LA, Leibner E, McKenney MG, et al. Randomized controlled clinical trial of point-of-care, limited ultrasonography for trauma in the emergency department: the first sonography outcomes assessment program trial. *Ann Emerg Med.* 2006;48(3):227–35.

7. Holmes JF, Kelley KM, Wootton-Gorges SL, et al. Effect of abdominal ultrasound on clinical care, outcomes, and resource use among children with blunt torso trauma: a randomized clinical trial. *JAMA.* 2017;317(22):2290–6.

8. Blackbourne LH, Soffer D, McKenney M, et al. Secondary ultrasound examination increases the sensitivity of the FAST exam in blunt trauma. *J Trauma.* 2004;57(5):934–8.

10 Clavicle Fracture! Simple! Not So Much!

Carrie DeHoff

A 15-year-old male presents to the emergency department (ED) via EMS following a motor vehicle collision. He was an unrestrained backseat passenger. By report the collision was a high-speed collision, with airbag deployment. Patient presented to the ED with complaint of difficulty swallowing as well as right clavicle and shoulder pain. He denies head injury and loss of consciousness. He denies chest pain, neck pain, back pain. Past medical history is noncontributory. He is on no regular medications. On physical examination, the patient is alert and oriented with a Glasgow Coma Scale of 15. He is handling his oral secretions normally. He has no midline spine tenderness. He has moderate swelling over the medial third of the right clavicle with swelling extending into the right anterior triangle of the neck. His extremities are nontender without deformity. He is neurovascularly intact in all extremities.

What do you do now?

PEDIATRIC SHOULDER INJURIES

The case presents a common presenting complaint in the ED. The differential for patients presenting with shoulder pain is broad and includes fractures (proximal humerus, clavicle, rib), physeal injuries, sprains of the acromioclavicular (AC) joint, and dislocations. Overall, rotator cuff injuries are uncommon in children. Labral tears are seen in traumatic injuries and in patients with shoulder instability. Stingers will be seen in adolescents most commonly, particularly athletes, and have associated transient neurologic symptoms. Given the patient's neck swelling and difficulty swallowing, vascular injury and intramuscular hematoma would also be on the differential. Bony lesions do not often present with pain unless associated with a pathologic fracture. Frozen shoulder, or adhesive capsulitis, although exquisitely painful, is typically seen remotely from the inciting injury or surgery, and is not common in the pediatric population.

ANATOMY OF THE SHOULDER

Anatomically, the clavicle is an S-shaped bone which acts as the anterior bony attachment for muscles as part of the shoulder suspensory complex. The clavicle sits on the anterior chest wall, situated between the sternum medially and the acromion process laterally. It is the first long bone to ossify, and one of the latest to fuse all growth plates. Ossification begins at 5 weeks gestational age, and the medial epiphysis is the last to ossify, typically fusing between 23 and 25 years of age. The majority of growth occurs at the medial physis. The middle third of the clavicle is the thinnest portion of the bone, making it most susceptible to fracture.

The history and physical exam findings can help differentiate the common sources of shoulder pain. Fractures typically present with a history of trauma directly associated with the onset of pain. The exception to this would be with pathologic fractures, which can occur in weakened bone with little to no trauma. A unicameral bone cyst (UBC) is usually the most common cause of pathological fracture in children with a bone lesion. However, the most common sites of pathological fractures due to UBC are the proximal humerus followed by the proximal femur.

The location of bony tenderness, along with the mechanism of injury provided can narrow the differential in patients presenting with shoulder pain. Examination of the shoulder should include inspection, palpation, range of motion, and neurovascular exams. Inspection looks at the symmetry of the injured shoulder when compared to the unaffected side. Physical exam findings suggestive of shoulder dislocation include a sulcus sign and deformity at the glenohumeral joint. In inferior dislocations, the arm is fixed in full abduction with the arm over the head.

Range of motion can be limited due to pain in the acute setting with traumatic injuries of the shoulder. In patients presenting with subacute pain, the location of pain, and provocative testing can help localize the source of the patients' symptoms. See table for shoulder tests.

Examination	Technique	Significance
Impingement/RTC		
Impingement sign	Passive FF beyond 90 degrees	pain = impingement
Hawkins	Passive FF 90 degrees and IR	pain = impingement
Jobe	Resisted pronation/FF 90 degrees	pain = supraspinatus
Drop-arm test	Maintain FF in plane of scapula	inability = supraspinatus
Liftoff test	Arm IR behind back	inability = subscapularis
Belly-push test	Elbow held anteriorly while applying abdominal pressure	inability = subscapularis
Instability		
Apprehension test	supine abd 90 degrees and ER	anterior instability
Relocation test	apprehension with posterior force to humeral head	relief = anterior instability
Load-and-shift test	Anterior/posterior force on humeral head	laxity vs. instability
Jerk test	posterior force, arm adducted and FF	clunk posterior subluxation

Examination	Technique	Significance
Sulcus sign	inferior force with arm at side	inferior laxity vs. instability
Labrum/Biceps		
Active compression test	10 degrees add, 90 FF, maximum pronation	SLAP
Anterior slide test	hand on hip, joint loaded	SLAP
Crank test	full abd humeral load, rotation	SLAP
Speed test	resisted FF in scapular plane	biceps tendinitis
Yerguson test	resisted supination	biceps tendinitis
Other		
Spurling test	lateral flexion, rotation, axial load	c-spine pathology/ radiculopathy
Wright's test	ext adb ER arm with neck rotated away	thoracic outlet

Source: Table adapted from *Miller's Review of Orthopedics.*

Clavicle fractures account for approximately 8%–15% of all childhood fractures, making it one of the most common fractures sustained in children. In infants, birth injury is the most common mechanism leading to a clavicle fracture. In all other age groups, clavicle fractures occur due to direct blow to the shoulder, whether from falls, sports injury and collisions, and motor vehicle accidents and those involving recreational vehicles. In adolescents, high-energy mechanisms increase in frequency, leading to more severe fracture patterns.

Clavicle fractures are classified anatomically. Clavicle shaft fractures involving the middle third are the most common, accounting for over 69%–85% of all clavicle fractures. Distal clavicle fractures are less common, accounting for 10%–21% of clavicle fractures. Medial third clavicle fractures account for 1%–5% of all clavicle fractures. Medial clavicle fractures are associated with high-energy mechanisms, particularly motor vehicle collisions; involvement of the sternoclavicular (SC) joint makes these injuries even more problematic.

Fracture patterns in pediatric clavicle fractures are also used to describe these injuries. Uncomplicated fracture patterns include greenstick fractures and simple fractures without significant displacement, shortening, or comminution. Uncomplicated fractures typically involve the medial third of the clavicle as well. Complicated fractures include comminuted, open, and significantly shortened and/or displaced fractures.

Pediatric acromioclavicular (AC) injuries are typically physeal injuries or occult fractures and not ligament injuries. Fractures and dislocations of the SC joint are unusual (less than 5% of traumatic injuries) but potentially devastating injuries in adolescents and young adults. Anterior fracture/dislocations are more common than posterior. Anterior fracture/dislocations are typically associated with a prominent and palpable medial clavicle. Posterior fracture/dislocations typically have more pain than anterior dislocations, and the injury is more likely to get overlooked due to subtle physical exam findings. Posterior dislocation can be associated with dysphagia and respiratory difficulties. Subtle findings such as ipsilateral upper extremity weakness, neck venous engorgement, or a diminished pulse can be seen. Posterior dislocations with severe displacement can present with a pneumothorax or shock from vascular compression.

Based on the patient in the scenario's history of significant trauma and difficulty swallowing and physical exam findings, including moderate swelling over the medial third of the right clavicle with swelling extending into the right anterior triangle of the neck, suspicion for a clavicle fracture and SC dislocation must be considered.

DIAGNOSIS

Imaging must now be considered. The standard imaging for an acute shoulder injury is 3 views of the shoulder. This will include an anterior–posterior (AP) view, a true AP of the shoulder (Grashey view), and a scapular Y view. Axillary views are necessary if dislocation is suspected. Focused imaging of the clavicle includes two views of the clavicle, which include an AP of the clavicle and a sunrise view which is angled 15 degrees cephalad.

Radiographs should be obtained in patients presenting with a traumatic injury to the shoulder. If pain is localized, imaging can be limited to the region of interest. Specialized views can help further clarify fracture patterns identified on initial views.

This patient had radiographs obtained, which revealed a displaced medial third clavicle fracture with dislocation of the SC joint (Figure 10.1). While clavicle fractures are quite common, this particular injury pattern is quite rare and seen primarily with high-energy mechanisms. Axial CT cuts are considered the gold standard to evaluate for dislocations.

In the patient from the scenario orthopedics was consulted for further management. CT scan of the chest and ultrasound were obtained to evaluate for underlying vascular injury.

Treatment

Treatment for uncomplicated clavicle fractures is typically nonoperative. In a survey completed by the Pediatric Orthopedic Society of North America, surgeons treated the vast majority of nondisplaced or angulated fractures nonoperatively. Use of a figure 8 harness or simple slings are the most common treatment modalities. Reported indications for emergent orthopedic consultation for operative management include markedly displaced fractures with compromised skin integrity, open fractures, concomitant vascular injury requiring repair, and compromise of the brachial plexus. More recently, there has been some support for operative management of middle third fractures with marked displacement (significant shortening >2 cm) specifically in adolescents.

There is variation in practice regarding follow-up care for simple clavicle fractures. Knowledge of community practice expectations is important, as many primary care clinics are willing and capable of providing the appropriate follow-up care for these injuries. Urgent orthopedic referral (within 2–3 days) may be considered for children/adolescents with significant shortening, given the current controversy.

Sternoclavicular dislocations require emergent orthopedic consultation. The treatment for anterior dislocations is nonoperative. Anterior dislocations can be reduced, though many are unstable even after reduction. A figure-of-eight brace may be used to hold the reduction. Posterior dislocations are treated urgently in the operating room with thoracic surgery on standby. Vascular injuries have been reported after reduction of the dislocation.

Uncomplicated clavicle fractures are rarely associated with other injuries (rarely vascular or brachial plexus) and the most frequent complication following nonoperative management, although rare, is nonunion. Fractures managed operatively may have hardware complications, and infections are complications associated with surgical intervention.

Acute complications associated with SC dislocations include great vessel and/or trachea injury, dyspnea, hoarseness, dysphagia. Additionally, traumatic pneumothorax, pneumomediastinum or tracheal stenosis can also occur. A tracheoesophageal fistula created by a missed posterior SC dislocation has been reported and resulted in death of the patient. Chronic dislocations have caused brachial plexopathies, exertional dyspnea, sepsis, SC joint arthritis, voice changes, and thoracic outlet syndrome. Potential hardware migration is a complication of operative treatment. The most common chronic complication is activity related pain.

CASE CONCLUSION

The patient was admitted for surgical fixation of his fracture dislocation. Cardiothoracic surgery was made aware of his injury and plan for surgical repair.

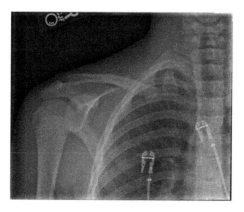

FIGURE 10.1. AP x-ray showing a medial third clavicle fracture with dislocation of the sternoclavicular joint

Further Reading

Shah RR, Kinder J, Peelman J, Moen TC, Sarwark J. Pediatric clavicle and acromioclavicular injuries. *J Pediatr Orthop.* 2010;30(2).S69–72.

Caird MS. Clavicle shaft fractures: are children little adults? *J Pediatr Orthop.* 2012;32:S1–4.

Adamich J, Howard A, Camp M. Do all clavicle fractures need to be managed by orthopedic surgeons? *Pediatr Emerg Care.* 2018;34(10):706–10.

Van der Meijden OA, Gaskill TR, Millett PJ. Treatment of clavicle fractures: current concepts review. *J Shoulder Elbow Surg.* 2012; 21:423–9.

Boutis K. Common pediatric fractures treated with minimal intervention. *Pediatr Emerg Care.* 2010;26(2):152–62.

Carry PM, Koonce R, Pan Z, Polousky JD. A survey of physician opinion adolescent midshaft clavicle fracture treatment preferences among POSNA members. *J Pediatr Orthop.* 2011;31(1):44–9.

Gausden EB, Fabricant PD. Management of clavicle fractures in adolescents. *JBJS Rev.* 2018;6(9):e4, 1–12.

Strauss BJ, Carey TP, Seabrook JA, Lim R. Pediatric clavicular fractures: assessment of fracture patterns and predictors of complicated outcome. *J Emerg Med.* 2012;4 (1):29–35.

McKee RC, Whelan DB, Schemitsch EH, McKee MD. Operative Versus Nonoperative Care of Displaced Midshaft Clavicle Fractures: A Meta-Analysis of Randomized Clinical Trials. *J Bone Joint Surg Am.* 2012;94:675–84.

11   I Kneed help!

Kristol Das

A 16-year-old previously healthy male presents with right knee pain following a fall off of his bike 7 days ago. He fell onto a concrete surface with the bike landing on top of him with his right knee closest to the ground. He denies hearing any pops or cracks at the time of injury. Immediately after the injury, he was diagnosed with a knee contusion at an urgent care. He returns due to continued knee pain and a clicking sensation while active. He trialed ibuprofen, ice, and rest at home with minimal improvement. He has no prior knee injuries and is sexually active with 2 female partners. His exam is notable for an antalgic gait favoring the left, a mild effusion, a midline patella, with pain localizing to the anterior patella in a band-like distribution. He has a negative Lachman's maneuver, posterior drawer test, and no patellar apprehension. He has 5/5 quadriceps strength and 2+ reflexes. Pain occurs with both resisted passive flexion and extension past 90 degrees.

What do you do now?

DIAGNOSIS

The differential diagnosis of knee pain after traumatic injury with direct trauma to the knee includes fracture of the patella, femur, or tibia; anterior cruciate ligament (ACL), posterior cruciate ligament (PCL), or meniscus sprain versus tear; and hematoma, effusion, or contusion. During evaluation, consideration should be given to structures above and below the knee and included in physical examination maneuvers assessing inspection, palpation, range of motion, and strength (Table 11.1). It is essential in any child with knee pain to do a careful and complete examination of the hip. This patient has a normal hip exam with full range of motion and no pain in the hip area.

Once injury is localized to the knee, several special maneuvers can be performed. To test the integrity of knee ligaments, use the Lachman's maneuver, posterior drawer test, and McMurray's test for the ACL, PCL, and meniscus, respectively. In the setting of significant knee swelling after knee trauma limiting examination, immobilize the knee and arrange follow-up in 1 week for re-examination if pain persists. In our patient, these maneuvers were not limited by swelling as he presented 1 week after the injury.

After a complete physical exam, consider the need for imaging. The Ottawa Knee Rules state that x-rays of the knee should be obtained in acute trauma with the presence of one of the following criteria: (1) tenderness at the head of the fibula, (2) isolated patellar tenderness, (3) inability to flex to 90 degrees, (4) inability to bear weight. This testing has high sensitivity and adequate specificity in children above 5 years old.[5] If any suspicion of patellar injury, 3 views (anterior–posterior [AP]/lateral/notch) should be obtained. In other cases, AP/lateral views are sufficient. As with physical exam maneuvers, consider imaging joints above and below the knee.

Due to persistent patellar pain as well as mild effusion, x-rays were obtained in this case and showed evidence of osteochondritis dissecans (OCD) that was later confirmed on MRI. OCD is a subchondral bone defect that can affect the surrounding articular cartilage. It can present after a single traumatic event, but typically presents more insidiously. The mechanism of this bone defect is not well understood. There may be a genetic component that predisposes the bone to traumatic versus vascular injury leading to osteochondral separation. Alternatively, repetitive microtrauma

TABLE 11.1. Knee Special Tests

	Features of a Positive Test	Sensitivity	Specificity
Lachman's *ACL*	- positive when absent endpoint to anterior displacement of tibia - **note**: higher sensitivity than anterior drawer test	0.86	0.91
McMurray's *medial and lateral meniscus*	- positive with "clicking sensation" with maneuver.	0.61	0.85
Wilson's Sign *medial femoral osteochondritis dissecans*	- positive with pain on internal rotation of tibia during knee extension and relief lateral tibial rotation - **note**: limited diagnostic utility	low	high
Posterior Drawer *PCL*	- Positive if increased posterior tibial displacement compared with uninvolved extremity.	Limited data	Limited data
Patellar Apprehension *patellar instability*	- Apprehension with lateral patellar movement suggestive of patellar instability	n/a	n/a

Sources: Carey JL, Shea K. AAOS clinical practice guideline: management of anterior cruciate ligament injuries: evidence-based guideline. *J Am Acad Orthopaed Surg.* 2015;23:32–53. doi:10.5435/JAAOS-D-15-00095.

Ostrowski JA. Accuracy of 3 diagnostic tests for anterior cruciate ligament tears. *J Athl Train.* 2006;41(1):120–1.

Smith BE, Thacker D, Crewesmith A, et al. Special tests for assessing meniscal tears within the knee: a systematic review and meta-analysis. *BMJ Evidence-Based Med.* 2015;20:88–97.

Conrad JM, Stanitski CL. Osteochondritis dissecans: Wilson's sign revisited. *Am J Sports Med.* 2003;31(5):777–8. doi:10.1177/0363546503010052301.

may lead to a stress reaction in the bone. Prior to the bike injury, our patient was an avid basketball player. Accordingly, one risk factor for OCD is participation in sports with repetitive impact. In addition, population-based cohort studies have shown that incidence in males is 4 times as high as in female patients and adolescents aged 12–19 years old had 3 times the risk of OCD as 6- to 11-year-old children.[4] Obesity is also a known risk factor.

In addition to typical knee examination maneuvers, Wilson's test is a special test to evaluate for OCD. A positive Wilson's test is defined as: pain with internally rotating the tibia during extension of the knee. There is relief of pain with tibial external rotation. Our patient had a positive Wilson's test. Due to the likely underlying intrinsic defect predisposing patients to these lesions, when a lesion is identified on one side, imaging should be obtained on the contralateral side to evaluate for bilateral defects. In cases of trauma or sports injury, MRI should be obtained for grading of injury as well as to rule out concomitant knee pathology such as articular cartilage or ligamentous injury.

Management depends on lesion stability and skeletal maturity. In unstable lesions where the osteochondral fragment is separate from parent bone, surgical management is likely necessary. In patients with open physes, lesions will often heal without surgery. These patients should be advised to avoid repetitive, high-impact activities and may benefit from knee immobilization and partial weight bearing until follow-up. Given the potential for lesion instability and need for surgical intervention, orthopedics consult or follow-up is indicated. This patient went on to have surgical correction due to the instability of the lesion and skeletal maturity.

KEY POINTS TO REMEMBER

- Obtain 3 views of the knee if any suspicion of patellar injury.
- Carefully examine the joints above (especially the hip) and below the knee in a patient with a chief complaint of knee pain.
- In OCD, orthopedics consultation/referral is indicated.
  Immediate referral for unstable lesions, within 6 months for stable lesions.

Further Reading

1. Bulloch B, Neto G, Plint A, et al. Validation of the Ottawa knee rule in children: a multicenter study. *Ann Emerg Med*. 2003;42(1):48–55. doi:10.1067/mem.2003.196.

2. Chambers HG, Shea KG, Carey JL. AAOS clinical practice guideline: diagnosis and treatment of osteochondritis dissecans. *Am Acad Orthopaed Surg*. 2011;19(5):307–9. doi:10.5435/00124635-201105000-00008.

3. Kessler JI, Jacobs JC, Cannamela PC, Shea KG, Weiss JM. Childhood obesity is associated with osteochondritis dissecans of the knee, ankle, and elbow in children and adolescents. *J Ped Orthopaed*. 2018;38(5):296–9. doi:10.1097/bpo.0000000000001158.

4. Kessler JI, Nikizad H, Shea KG, Jacobs JC, Ishkhanian RM, Weiss J. The demographics, epidemiology, and incidence of progression to surgery of osteochondritis dissecans of the knee in children and adolescents. *Orthopaed J Sports Med*. 2013;1(4_suppl). doi:10.1177/2325967113s00075.

5. Vijayasankar D, Boyle AA, Atkinson P. Can the Ottawa knee rule be applied to children? A systematic review and meta-analysis of observational studies. *Emerg Med J*. 2009;26(4):250–3. doi:10.1136/emj.2008.063131.

12 Let's Do the Twist

Laurie Malia and Joni E. Rabiner

A 10-year-old previously healthy male presented to the emergency department with ankle pain and swelling after an injury today. He endorsed that he was in gym class playing basketball and twisted his ankle while attempting a layup and he felt a "pop." The ankle is now painful, swollen, and he is unable to ambulate. He denies any numbness or tingling. His vital signs are unremarkable. Physical examination is notable for swelling to the right lateral ankle, with point tenderness to palpation over the posterior lateral malleolus and distal fibula. There is decreased range of motion of the ankle but he is able to wiggle his toes. He has 2+ dorsalis pedis pulses, capillary refill is less than 2 seconds, and sensation is intact.

What do you do now?

DISCUSSION

In this previously healthy boy with acute onset of ankle pain and swelling after injury, the differential diagnosis includes ankle fracture and ankle sprain, with ankle sprain being significantly more common than ankle fracture. However, it is important to differentiate fractures from sprains, as fractures may occur in up to 20% of ankle injuries and require immobilization and/or surgery to prevent morbidity. In addition, this 10-year-old boy has open physes, which may require special consideration when evaluating an ankle injury in a child.[1]

Following pain control, the next step is to determine if imaging with a 3-view x-ray of the ankle is indicated, as x-ray is the standard of care to evaluate for fracture at the ankle. Do radiographs always need to be performed when a pediatric patient presents with an ankle injury? Both the Ottawa Ankle Rules and the Low Risk Ankle Rule are clinical decision rules that have been validated in children and help guide which patients require radiographic imaging (Table 12.1). The Ottawa Ankle Rules are used to identify patients at low risk of ankle fracture that do not require

TABLE 12.1. **Comparison of Ottawa Ankle Rules and Low Risk Ankle Rules**

	Ottawa Ankle Rules	Low Risk Ankle Rule
Age	>5 years	3 years–16 years
Sensitivity[1,9]	98.5%	100%
Specificity[1,9]	8%–47%	68%
Rule	**x-ray of the ankle is NOT indicated** if the patient does NOT have pain near either malleoli plus does NOT have: · Bone tenderness at the posterior tip of the lateral malleolus · Bone tenderness at the posterior tip of the medial malleolus · Unable to weight bear at the time of injury and when being evaluated	**x-ray of the ankle is NOT indicated** if: · Injury is < 3 days old AND · Tenderness or swelling isolated to the distal fibula and/or adjacent lateral ligaments distal to the anterior joint line

x-ray imaging. If a patient does not have pain isolated to the posterior edge or tip of the medial or lateral malleolus, or if the patient is able to bear weight after the injury or in the emergency department for 4 steps, then the patient is low risk for fracture and does not require radiographic imaging. The Low Risk Ankle Rule can be applied to children ages 3 to 16 years, up to 72 hours after an ankle injury. Per the Low Risk Ankle Rule, if there is pain isolated to the distal fibula and/or adjacent lateral ligaments distal to the tibial anterior joint line, then the child is low risk for significant fracture and does not require x-ray imaging. Applying this rule, however, may miss distal fibular avulsion fractures or nondisplaced Salter-Harris type I or II fractures, which are considered low risk fractures and can be managed conservatively (splinting and crutches). The Ottawa Ankle Rules and the Low Risk Ankle Rule have been shown to reduce radiography in children by up to 25%, without missing clinically significant fractures.

Point-of-care ultrasound performed by emergency physicians has shown potential as a screening test for ankle fracture in patients with ankle injuries. Studies with adult patients have shown both high sensitivity and specificity in the diagnosis of ankle fractures and that using ultrasound as a screening test can decrease overall radiographs needed in the evaluation of ankle injuries.[2] However, there is no data yet for pediatrics and patients with open growth plates.

Pediatric patients with open physes need to be evaluated and managed differently than adults. In children with open growth plates, the Salter-Harris nomenclature can be used to describe fractures involving the physis, with fractures graded on a scale from I to V.[3] The growth of the bone occurs at the physis and can be prone to injury. If not appropriately treated with immobilization, growth plate injuries can cause morbidity including asymmetric bone growth, growth failure, or range of motion limitations. A Salter-Harris type I fracture is a fracture through the physis, and a high clinical suspicion must be maintained in the evaluation for a nondisplaced Salter-Harris type I fracture, as they most often have normal x-ray imaging. With Salter-Harris type I fractures, the patient will have pain with palpation over the growth plate of the long-bone. However, in a recent study of children with lateral ankle trauma and clinically suspected Salter-Harris type I injuries, MRI showed that Salter-Harris type I distal fibula fractures are exceedingly rare (3%), with ligamentous injuries, occult fibular avulsion fractures, and bone contusions occurring significantly more frequently.[4] Salter-Harris type II, III, and IV fractures will be identified by radiographic imaging. A Salter-Harris type II fracture is a break through the physis including the metaphysis, type III is a fracture through the physis and involving the epiphysis, and type IV is a fracture that crosses through the epiphysis, physis, and metaphysis. A Salter-Harris type V fracture is a crush fracture of the physis that occurs with more traumatic mechanisms of injury and may or may not be visualized on x-rays (Figure 12.1).

Management for ankle sprains usually involves bracing with an ace wrap or air cast with early mobilization and weight bearing as tolerated, crutches temporarily as needed for inability to bear weight, and follow-up with either a pediatrician or an orthopedist for persistent symptoms. Most patients should be able to walk without pain in 1–3 weeks.[5]

For fibular fractures, Salter-Harris type I and II fractures and avulsion fractures of the distal fibula immobilization may be accomplished with an air cast, removable ankle brace, or plaster or fiber-glass splint.[6,7] Patients should remain non-weight-bearing until the pain improves and follow-up with orthopedics within 1 week, with most patients making a full recovery within 6–12 weeks. Salter-Harris type III, IV, and V fractures of the fibula are uncommon but require orthopedic consultation for management and follow-up.

For tibial fractures, Salter-Harris type I and II tibial fractures that are nondisplaced can be immobilized using a posterior leg splint and crutches with orthopedic follow-up within 1 week.[8] Nondisplaced Salter-Harris type III fractures should be evaluated by an orthopedist but are typically managed by placement of a long leg cast for 4 to 6 weeks. Salter-Harris type IV tibial fractures, also known as triplane fractures, require orthopedic consultation and typically a CT scan to evaluate the degree of displacement and to plan management. Salter-Harris type V fractures of the tibia require urgent orthopedic evaluation and management in the emergency department. Any displaced fractures involving either the fibula or tibia also require urgent orthopedic consultation.

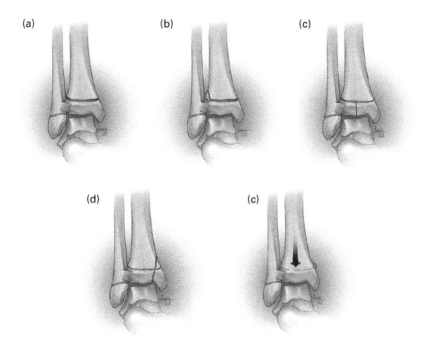

(a)   (b)   (c)

(d)   (c)

FIGURE 12.1. Salter Harris Classification

As for our patient, since he is unable to bear weight both immediately after the injury and in the emergency department, and has pain to palpation over the posterior lateral malleolus, he is not low risk for fracture and requires x-ray imaging per the Ottawa Ankle Rules. He is, however, low risk for fracture per the Low Risk Ankle Rule. The decision is made to obtain radiographic imaging, which is negative for fracture, and he is given ibuprofen for his pain and ice for his swelling.

What do you do now?

Pain following an ankle injury with normal radiographs can result from ligament, muscle, or tendon strains or from Salter-Harris type I injuries in children with open physes. On re-evaluation after pain control, our patient is able to ambulate in the emergency department. He is diagnosed with a likely ankle sprain given his improvement in pain and ability to ambulate and the low likelihood of a Salter-Harris type I fracture of the distal fibula, and he is given an aircast for bracing. He is counseled to use RICE for the next week: rest with ambulation as tolerated, ice for swelling, compression with aircast for support, and elevation for swelling. He will continue ibuprofen as needed for pain, and he will follow up with his pediatrician in 1 week if he has persistent pain or difficulty with ambulation.

KEY POINTS TO REMEMBER

· Clinical decision rules have been validated in children to determine who is at low risk for significant fracture and may not need radiographic evaluation for ankle injury.

· Children with open physes may have Salter-Harris type I fractures with normal x-rays; however, this has been shown to be exceedingly rare for distal fibular injuries.

· Nondisplaced Salter-Harris type I and II fractures of the distal fibula and tibia can be managed with immobilization and out-patient orthopedic follow-up within 1 week.

· Salter Harris III, IV, and V fractures of the fibula and tibia and all displaced fractures require orthopedic consultation.

Further Reading

1. Dowling S, Spooner CH, Liang Y, et al. Accuracy of Ottawa ankle rules to exclude fractures of the ankle and midfoot in children: a meta-analysis. *Acad Emerg Med.* 2009;16:277.

2. Hedelin H, Goksor L, Karlsson J, et al. Ultrasound-assisted triage of ankle trauma can decrease the need for radiographic imaging. *Am J Emerg Med.* 2013;31:1686–9.

3. Tandberg D, Sherbring M. A mnemonic for Salter-Harris classification. *Am J Emerg Med.* 1999;17:321.

4. Boutis K, Plint A, Stimec J. Radiographic-negative lateral ankle injuries in children occult growth plate fracture or sprain? *JAMA Pediatrics.* 2016;170(1):e154114.

5. Miller TL, Skalak T. Evaluation and treatment recommendations for acute injuries to the ankle syndesmosis without associated fracture. *Sports Med.* 2014;44(2):179.

6. Boutis K, Willan AR, Babyn P, et al. A randomized controlled trial of a removable brace versus casting in children with low-risk ankle fractures. *Pediatrics.* 2007;119(6):e1256.

7. Barnett PL, Lee MH, Oh L, et al. Functional outcome after air-stirrup ankle brace or fiberglass backslap for pediatric low-risk-ankle fractures: a randomized observer-blinded controlled trial. *Pediatr Emerg Care.* 2012;28(8):745.

8. Marsh JS, Daigneault JP. Ankle injuries in the pediatric population. *Curr Opin Pediatr.* 2000;12(1):52.

9. Boutis K, Komar L, Jaramillo D, et al. Sensitivity of a clinical examination to predict need for radiography in children with ankle injuries: a prospective study. *Lancet.* 2001;358:2118–21.

13 What Goes Up and Up— Comes Down and Down

Ajay K. Puri and Philipp J. Underwood

A 13-year-old male with no prior medical issues presents to your emergency department (ED) complaining of right ankle pain after landing on his right leg after jumping off a swing at the top of its arc. This occurred just prior to coming to the ED. He has been unable to bear weight on his right lower extremity due to pain and noticed his ankle is swollen. He complains of no other injuries. His vital signs are normal. He appears uncomfortable. His right ankle is swollen with tenderness to palpation over the medial malleolus without any overlying skin changes. His compartments are soft to palpation. Sensation to pinprick in his foot is intact. He is able to wiggle his toes, with range of motion around his ankle limited by pain. Capillary refill is less than 2 seconds in his toes and a strong posterior tibial pulse is palpated.

What do you do now?

INTRODUCTION

The patient has radiographs of his foot and ankle taken. The x-rays of his foot are normal. An x-ray of his ankle is displayed in Figure 13.1.

One of the main differences between the skeleton of an adult and a growing pediatric patient is the presence of a physis, also known as a growth plate. It refers to a group of proliferative cartilaginous cells located between the epiphysis distally and metaphysis proximally. It is the weakest part of the child's skeleton, and is particularly susceptible to injury or fracture during periods of rapid growth, as in adolescence. Ligaments in children are often stronger than the integrity of the physis, hence injuries that would cause a sprain in adults may cause a physeal injury in children. The Salter-Harris (SH) system is the most frequently used approach to describe these patterns of injuries. It ranges from type I to V. Higher numbers are associated with greater chances of growth arrest, or premature physeal closure (PPC), and misalignment. Hence, management of these injuries primarily focuses on successful reduction to prevent PPC and deformity with appropriate immobilization and, if necessary, operative intervention. This chapter describes diagnosis of SH fractures, subsequent emergency management of each injury pattern, and the urgency with which an orthopedic surgeon should be involved in the care of the patient.

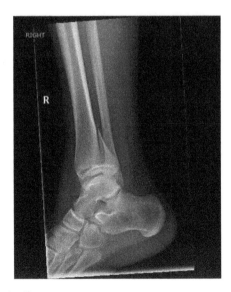

FIGURE 13.1.   Lateral ankle x-ray.

EPIDEMIOLOGY

The physis is involved in up to 35% of all pediatric fractures. The most frequent sites of physeal injury are the distal radius (30%–60% of cases), distal tibia, and distal fibula. Adolescents are the most susceptible age group. Physeal injuries are twice as common in males compared to females due to the longer period the physis of their bones remain open and a higher incidence of musculoskeletal injuries in males.

PHYSEAL STRUCTURE

To understand why physeal injuries carry a worse prognosis with higher SH classification numbers, a general understanding of physeal structure is helpful. The physis consists of 4 zones. In distal to proximal order from the epiphysis they are; the germinal zone, the proliferative zone, the hypertrophic zone, and the zone of provisional calcification. The hypertrophic zone is the most common site of fractures within the physis for two reasons; it is avascular and it has very little extracellular cartilage to support it. Arterial blood supply to the physis is primarily from the epiphysial side through the epiphyseal artery, with secondary supply coming from the metaphyseal side through nutrient vessels. These vessels do not penetrate down to the hypertrophic zone. However, disruption of the epiphysis, and consequently primary arterial supply to the physis along with the germinal and proliferative layers, in SH III and IV fractures explains why these fractures have a worse prognosis.

SALTER-HARRIS I AND V

SH I injuries are transections of the physis on the horizontal plane. These mostly occur through the hypertrophic zone. These fractures have a less than 1% chance of PPC, as the germinal and proliferative zones are relatively unaffected and vascular injury is unlikely. These injuries mostly occur in infants, and the mechanism typically involves an avulsion, shearing, or torsion movement that leads to separation of the physis. They only account for 6% of physeal injuries. Despite this, the presence of an SH I injury should be suspected in any child presenting with a joint injury with negative plain films due to frequently normal-appearing radiographs. These fractures heal rapidly, within 2–3 weeks of the initial injury.

In stark contrast, SH V fractures are typically "crush" injuries, frequently sustained in the knee or ankle. The mechanism involved is a severe abduction or adduction injury that transmits high compressive forces over the physis. This compression directly injures the germinal and proliferative zones and has an almost 100% rate of PPC as it, by definition, prematurely closes the physis. SH V fractures fortunately have a low incidence, constituting less than 1% of physeal injuries. Similar to SH I fractures, these injuries are often not detected on x-rays until growth abnormalities occur.

We grouped SH I and V fractures together because their diagnosis typically relies on a thorough history and physical examination in contrast to plain films, as radiographs for both these fractures are usually normal. The ED management of both injuries is also typically the same, with immobilization and orthopedic follow-up. The reason for immobilization is 2-fold; for resolution of pain and for prevention of PPC. Prompt immobilization in Salter-Harris I injuries reduces the duration of tenderness at the joint possibly from weeks to 5–7 days. When radiographs are normal or display an SH I injury, these patients should be immobilized in-plane with a splint and should be followed by an orthopedist as an outpatient for serial radiographs to evaluate for PPC. Intermittent icing and elevation can ease pain and discomfort. It is imperative that parents be counseled that immobilization is for the worst-case scenario and that their child likely will not have PPC, however this can only be determined on serial radiographs as an outpatient.

An important caveat is that when SH V fractures *are* detected on x-rays, orthopedic consultation is warranted given the poor prognosis of these injuries. Since the lower extremities are typically involved, patients are usually casted and kept non-weight-bearing.

SALTER-HARRIS II

SH II fractures transect the growth plate and extend into the metaphysis leading to a metaphyseal bone fragment known as a Thurston-Holland fragment. They account for the majority of physeal fractures at approximately

75%. These fractures also do not affect the germinal or proliferative layer and hence do not typically lead to vascular disruption to the growth plate. They also have a low risk of PPC at a rate only slightly higher than SH I fractures. The exceptions are physeal fractures of the lower extremity such as those involving the tibia and fibula. These carry a PPC rate up to 40%. Surgical reduction of these fractures does not seem to improve these rates and may paradoxically increase the need for subsequent surgeries. In the ED, it is sufficient to reduce these fractures as effectively as possible and ensure close orthopedic follow-up.

Nondisplaced fractures are treated with immobilization with a splint or cast and to be followed up by an orthopedist, similar to SH I fractures. Displaced fractures should undergo a closed reduction and subsequent immobilization. These would ideally be reduced up to 10–15 degrees of angulation in the distal radius, and with less than 2 mm displacement at the ankle and knee with non-weight-bearing status.

Where this may not be achieved, Stutz et al. recommends a relative indication of pinning or operative intervention only in fractures of greater than 30 degrees angulation or more than 50% displacement in distal radius SH II fractures deferring to surgeon preference in specific instances due to the high remodeling capacity of the distal radius. Russo et al. divided patients with distal tibial SH II fractures into 4 categories; up to 2 mm displacement treated with a long-leg cast, 2–4 mm treated with a long leg cast, 2–4 mm treated with open reduction and internal fixation (ORIF), and fractures more than 4 mm treated with ORIF. There was no significantly different rate of PPC in the operative groups versus the nonoperative groups. They recommend all SH II fractures of the distal tibia be treated with closed reduction and nonsurgical treatment without evidence of a gross deformity. We recommend that any decision with regard to disposition of a suboptimal reduction be made in conjunction with an orthopedic surgeon, particularly with older children, as they have less time to remodel their bones. Furthermore, these fractures may be difficult to reduce owing to entrapment of the periosteum or muscle between fracture fragments effectively physically blocking successful reduction. In these instances, eventual surgical exploration may be required to remove entrapped material before appropriate reduction. Moreover, any rotational deformity needs to be reduced.

SALTER-HARRIS III AND IV

SH III fractures are intraarticular fractures of the epiphysis with extension through the hypertrophic layer of the physis. These fractures are rare, and account for only 8%–10% of physeal fractures. The prognosis is good, but more guarded than SH I or II injuries. This is due to the possible disruption of blood supply from the epiphysis and due to the fracture extending through the germinal and proliferative cell layers in the physis. Larger degrees of displacement correspond to an increased probability of vascular disruption and consequent PPC.

SH IV fractures also represent intra-articular fractures of the epiphysis and into the physis, however the fracture line continues into the metaphysis and exits through a metaphyseal segment. These injuries account for approximately 10% of physeal injuries. They are typically seen in medial malleolus fractures of the ankle and lateral condyle separation in distal humerus fractures. Similar to SH III, blood supply may be disrupted, leading to PPC.

SH III and SH IV fractures require orthopedic consultation preferably in the ED as they are intra-articular and therefore frequently require surgical intervention to achieve near-perfect alignment of the articular surface to prevent PPC, premature cartilage wear, and arthritis. These fractures typically require ORIF and immobilization as the standard treatment.

ADDITIONAL CONSIDERATIONS WITH REDUCTION OF SALTER-HARRIS FRACTURES

A successful reduction can be facilitated with administration of effective conscious sedation with effective pain management. Effective sedation leads to increased patient, provider, and parental satisfaction while facilitating improved rates of successful fracture reduction. Children are often inadequately treated for their fracture pain in the ED, hence providers need to ensure this is a priority during their ED stay. Migita et al. compared the combination of ketamine (for sedation) and midazolam (for anxiolysis) to the combinations of fentanyl-midazolam and propofol-fentanyl for the purposes of pediatric fracture reduction. They found ketamine-midazolam had the lowest rate of adverse events. We suggest hematoma blocks or regional nerve blocks also be used in appropriate instances.

Multiple attempts at a closed reduction should ideally be avoided. It is theorized that repeat attempts at a closed reduction could further damage an already injured physis, and may contribute to PPC. However, this has not been demonstrated in the literature.

After a successful reduction, immobilization with splinting in the emergency department for SH I and SH II fractures is sufficient until orthopedic follow-up is soon established. Dittmer et al. found with reduced displaced fractures involving the pediatric forearm, a sugar-tong splint is as effective as a cast immobilization with regard to rates of loss of reduction. To our knowledge, this has not been investigated with reduced displaced fractures of the lower extremity.

COMPLICATIONS

While much of the focus surrounding SH fractures centers on the primary complication of PPC, pediatric patients with physeal fractures still need to be evaluated for standard complications of fractures.

Neurological and vascular compromise distal to the fracture need to be evaluated. Any evidence of neurovascular compromise associated with a fracture requires urgent closed reduction and orthopedic surgery evaluation for possible additional percutaneous pinning or open reduction.

Any evidence of neurovascular compromise needs to be differentiated from compartment syndrome. While rare in physeal injuries, this can be evaluated by measuring compartment pressures with a Stryker needle. It is imperative to measure compartment pressures away from the fracture site, where pressures will invariably be elevated. If pressures are elevated, a fasciotomy is necessary.

DIAGNOSIS

The patient is diagnosed with a displaced SH IV fracture of the distal tibia. He is determined to not have neurovascular compromise or signs of compartment syndrome or an open fracture. Orthopedic surgery is consulted and a closed reduction is performed under conscious sedation with 1 mg/kg of ketamine. The patient has a normal repeat neurovascular exam and is placed in a long-leg cast for immobilization. A postreduction x-ray is deemed satisfactory (seen in Figure 13.2). He is scheduled to follow up with a pediatric orthopedic surgeon in the next week for operative evaluation.

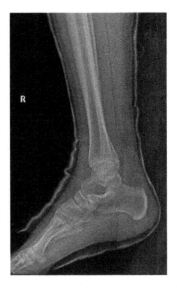

FIGURE 13.2. Lateral ankle x-ray after successful closed reduction and casting.

KEY POINTS TO REMEMBER

· If the diagnosis of a sprain or a strain is being entertained in a pediatric patient, the clinician should question why this does not represent an SH I fracture.

· SH I and SH II fractures are typically treated with closed reduction and immobilization with orthopedic follow-up.

· SH III, IV, and V fractures warrant orthopedic consultation in the ED when diagnosed.

· Adequate pain control, sedation, and anxiolysis are paramount to a successful reduction.

· While growth plate arrest dominates much of the conversation regarding complications of Salter-Harris fractures, be mindful of other complications of fractures such as neurovascular compromise and compartment syndrome.

Further Reading

1. Mallick A, Prem H. Physeal injuries in children. *Surgery (Oxford).* 2017;35(1): 10–17. doi:10.1016/j.mpsur.2016.10.008.
2. Jones C, Wolf M, Herman M. Acute and chronic growth plate injuries. *Pediatr Rev.* 2017;38(3):129–38. doi:10.1542/pir.2015-0160.
3. Perron A, Miller M, Brady W. Orthopedic pitfalls in the ED: pediatric growth plate injuries. *Am J Emerg Med.* 2002;20(1):50–4. doi:10.1053/ajem.2002.30096.
4. Stutz C, Mencio G. Fractures of the distal radius and ulna: metaphyseal and physeal injuries. *J Pediatr Orthopaed.* 2010;30:S85–9. doi:10.1097/bpo.0b013e3181c9c17a.
5. Asad W, Younis M, Ahmed A, Ibrahim T. Open versus closed treatment of distal tibia physeal fractures: a systematic review and meta-analysis. *Eur J Orthopaed Surg Traumatol.* 2017;28(3):503–9. doi:10.1007/s00590-017-2062-1.
6. Russo F, Moor M, Mubarak S, Pennock A. Salter-Harris II fractures of the distal tibia. *J Ped Orthopaed.* 2013;33(5):524–9. doi:10.1097/bpo.0b013e3182880279.
7. Migita R, Klein E, Garrison M. Sedation and analgesia for pediatric fracture reduction in the emergency department. *Arch Pediatr Adolesc Med.* 2006;160(1):46. doi:10.1001/archpedi.160.1.46.
8. Dittmer A, Molina D, Jacobs C, Walker J, Muchow R. Pediatric forearm fractures are effectively immobilized with a sugar-tong splint following closed reduction. *J Pediatr Orthopaed.* 2019;39(4):e245–7. doi:10.1097/bpo.0000000000001291.
9. Leary J, Handling M, Talerico M, Yong L, Bowe J. Physeal fractures of the distal tibia. *J Pediatr Orthopaed.* 2009;29(4):356–61. doi:10.1097/bpo.0b013e3181a6bfe8.

14 Where Do These Puzzle Pieces Go?

Mir Raza and Lara Reda

A 7-year-old girl is brought to the ED for left elbow pain after a fall while ice skating 1 hour ago. She has no history of head trauma, does not take any anticoagulants and has no other injuries. Patient does not have any medical problems or prior surgeries, and her immunizations are up to date. Vital signs are: heart rate 96 bpm, blood pressure 95/55, pulse oximetry 99% on room air, respiration 20 breaths per minute, temperature 98°F. Examination is notable for a well-appearing but anxious girl who is not moving her left arm. The left elbow is swollen with decreased active and passive range of motion and bony tenderness over the distal humerus. There is full active and passive range of motion at left shoulder and wrist. Capillary refill at the fingers of the left hand is less than 2 seconds, radial and ulnar pulses are 2+. Sensation is normal at left upper extremity. The remainder of physical exam is normal. You get an elbow radiograph (Figures 14.1 and 14.2). Are any of those pieces fractures?

What do you do now?

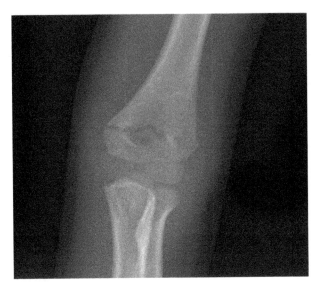

FIGURE 14.1. AP radiograph of the elbow (case courtesy of A.Prof Frank Gaillard, Radiopaedia. org, rID: 10342).

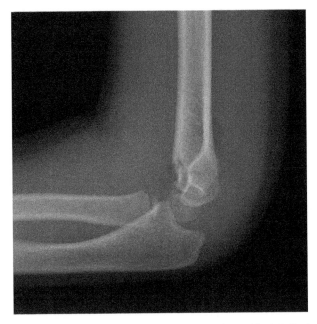

FIGURE 14.2. Lateral radiograph of the elbow (case courtesy of A.Prof Frank Gaillard, Radiopaedia.org, rID: 10342).

INTRODUCTION AND EPIDEMIOLOGY

Pediatric elbow injuries are very common and elbow fractures make up about 10% of all fractures in the pediatric patient population. The most common pediatric elbow fractures in descending order are: supracondylar humeral fracture, lateral condyle fracture, medial epicondyle fracture, radial head fracture, and radial neck fracture. Knowledge of how to interpret pediatric elbow x-rays, as well as knowledge of common injures, is essential to the correct assessment and management of these patients.

SIGNS, SYMPTOMS, AND DIFFERENTIAL DIAGNOSIS

Patients with elbow fractures typically have a history of falling on an outstretched hand, or direct trauma to the elbow. Most patients with elbow fractures have swelling at the site of the injury and an inability to move the affected joint. Apart from fractures of the elbow, other diagnosis to be considered include radial head subluxation (nursemaid's elbow), medial epicondyle apophysitis (little leaguer's elbow), and an elbow dislocation.

A good neurovascular physical exam needs to be performed to make sure there isn't any compromise. The vascular exam consists of checking the brachial and radial pulses, and checking capillary refill time. The neurological exam consists of checking the function of the median, radial, and ulnar nerves. Pediatric patients can be challenging, especially with a painful elbow injury. One way to get a good motor exam is to have the child make the hand gestures of "rock, paper, scissors" and "A-Ok" hand gestures. The median nerve allows for finger flexion, as in the "rock" hand gesture. The radial nerve allows for extension of the wrist and metacarpophalangeal joints, as in the "paper" hand gesture. The anterior interosseous nerve (a branch of the median nerve) allows for thumb flexion at the interphalangeal joint and flexion of the index finger at the distal interphalangeal joint, as in the "A-Ok" hand gesture. The ulnar nerve allows for extension of the wrist and metacarpophalangeal joints, as in the "paper" hand gesture. Nerve damage can also be detected by sensory changes across the dermatome map.

TECHNIQUES TO INTERPRET PEDIATRIC ELBOW PLAIN FILMS

Interpreting a pediatric elbow radiograph can be difficult and requires a systematic approach. First, make sure the elbow alignment is correct. On a lateral radiograph of the elbow, you should be able to make an imaginary figure "8" at the distal humerus. Second, check to see if the ossification centers are present in the correct position (Table 14.1 and Figure 14.3). The ossification centers appear in a predictable order and can be remembered by the acronym *CRITOE*.

Third, look for fat pads. Anterior fat pads may be normally visualized. If anterior fat pads are larger than normal they can appear as a boat sail or a "sail sign." Posterior fat pads visualized on radiographs are always abnormal and indicate an underlying elbow effusion.

Fourth, check for normal alignment using the anterior humeral line and radiocapitellar line. When an imaginary line is drawn from the anterior humerus, it should intersect the middle to anterior third of the capitellum (if it does not then a supracondylar fracture might be present). If an imaginary line is drawn from the middle of the radial neck, it should always intersect the capitellum (if it does not then a radial head dislocation might be present) (Figure 14.4).

Lastly, look at the bony cortex of the distal humerus, radius, and ulnar bones to evaluate any irregularities that might suggest a fracture.

TABLE 14.1. **Age at Which Ossification Centers Are Visible on X-Ray and Age When They Fuse**

Ossification Center	Approximate Age (in Years) at Ossification (on X-Ray)	Age (in Years) at Fusion (on X-Ray)
Capitellum	1	12
Radial Head	3	15
Internal/Medial Epicondyle	5	17
Trochlea	7	12
Olecranon	9	15
External/Lateral Epicondyle	11	12

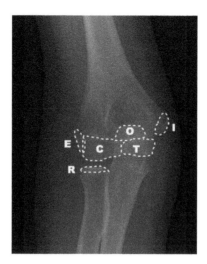

FIGURE 14.3. Normal AP elbow radiograph of an 11-year-old with all 6 ossification centers (case courtesy of Dr Andrew Dixon, Radiopaedia.org, rID: 20908).

DIAGNOSIS

The 7-year-old child in this case has a supracondylar fracture. The capitellum, radial head, internal epicondyle, and trochlea ossification centers can be

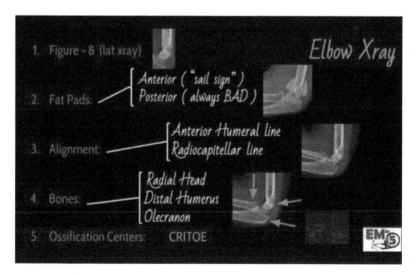

FIGURE 14.4. Systematic approach to interpreting pediatric elbow x-ray (courtesy of Dr Anna Pickens).

noted, which indicate the child is at least 7 years old. When the anterior humeral line is drawn, it does not intersect the middle to anterior third of the capitellum, indicating a supracondylar fracture. Supracondylar bony irregularities are also noted and consistent with a mildly posteriorly displaced supracondylar humeral fracture.

EMERGENCY DEPARTMENT MANAGEMENT AND TREATMENT

Supracondylar fractures are managed based on the neurovascular status of the affected extremity and based on the degree of displacement of the fracture. If there is any vascular compromise distal to the fracture site, an emergent bedside closed reduction needs to be performed by an orthopedic surgeon who should then emergently take the patient to the operating room for definitive surgical management. If there is any suspicion of compartment syndrome or if there is an open elbow fracture then emergent surgical management is needed.

Supracondylar fractures are classified according the Gartland Classification system (Table 14.2).

Gartland type I fractures that are neurovascularly intact can be managed by the emergency department provider using a long-arm splint and outpatient orthopedics follow-up within a week. Gartland type II and III fractures require an urgent orthopedics consult for management. There is practice variability among orthopedists on whether Gartland Type II and III fractures require surgical management (open or closed reduction and percutaneous pinning) or nonoperative management with a cast. However, most Gartland Type II and III fractures with neurological (motor or sensory) deficits are managed surgically.

It should be noted that humeral fractures are commonly associated with forearm fractures, so radiographs of the forearm should also be obtained.

TABLE 14.2. **Gartland Classification System**

Gartland Type I	Gartland Type II	Gartland Type III
Nondisplaced fracture	Displaced fracture with an intact posterior periosteum	Displaced fracture with disrupted anterior and posterior periosteum.

· 10% of all fractures in the pediatric patient population involve the elbow.

· To get a good neurological exam of the upper extremity have the child make the hand gestures of "rock, paper, scissors" and "A-Ok" to test the motor function of the median nerve, radial nerve, and ulnar nerve and anterior interosseous nerve, respectively.

· Systematic approach to interpret pediatric plain films: check alignment → check ossification centers → look for fat pads → draw the radiocapitellar line and the anterior humeral line → check for bony abnormalities.

· Posterior fat pads are always abnormal.

· Supracondylar fractures almost always require an emergent orthopedics consult unless patient has a Gartland type I fracture and is neurovascularly intact.

Further Reading

1. DeFroda SF, et al. Radiographic evaluation of common pediatric elbow injuries. *Orthop Rev (Pavia)*. 2017;9(1):7030.

2. Alton TB, et al. Classifications in brief: the Gartland classification of supracondylar humerus fractures. *Clin Orthopaed Relat Res.* 2015;473(2):738–41. www.ncbi.nlm.nih.gov/pmc/articles/PMC4294919/.

3. Abzug JM, Herman MJ. Management of supracondylar humerus fractures in children: current concepts. *J Am Acad Orthop Surg.* 2012;20(2):69–77. doi: 10.5435/JAAOS-20-02-069. www.ncbi.nlm.nih.gov/pubmed/22302444.

4. Ryan L. Elbow anatomy and radiographic diagnosis of elbow fracture in children. *UpToDate.* www.uptodate.com/contents/elbow-anatomy-and-radiographic-diagnosis-of-elbow-fracture-in-children?search=pediatric%2Belbow%2Bfracture&source=search_result&selectedTitle=1~150&usage_type=default&display_rank=1.

5. Ryan L. Evaluation and management of supracondylar fractures in children. *UpToDate.* www.uptodate.com/contents/evaluation-and-management-of-supracondylar-fractures-in-children?search=pediatric%2Belbow%2Bfracture&source=search_result&selectedTitle=4~150&usage_type=default&display_rank=4#H38.

6. Horeczko T. Pediatric elbow injuries. *Pediatric Emergency Playbook*, March 6, 2017. pemplaybook.org/podcast/pediatric-elbow-injuries/.

7. Pickens A. Elbow xray interpretation. *EM in 5*, June 19, 2015, emin5.com/2014/11/10/elbow-xray-interpretation/.

8. Supracondylar fracture—pediatric. *Orthobullets*. www.orthobullets.com/pediatrics/4007/supracondylar-fracture--pediatric.

9. Jones J. Pediatric elbow radiograph (an approach) | radiology reference article. *Radiopaedia Blog RSS*. radiopaedia.org/articles/paediatric-elbow-radiograph-an-approach?lang=us.

10. Gaillard F. Supracondylar fracture | radiology case. *Radiopaedia Blog RSS*, radiopaedia.org/cases/supracondylar-fracture-4?lang=us.

15 Why Am I Banged Up?

Shilpa Hari, Dana Kaplan, and Isabel A. Barata

A 3-month-old female presents to the ED with her father for nasal congestion and cough that has been occurring for 3 days. Father states she has been afebrile, feeding at baseline, with normal urine output. Her 5-year-old brother has similar symptoms and goes to daycare. She was born premature at 34 weeks via vaginal delivery and was admitted to the neonatal ICU, where her course was uncomplicated. She has no other past medical or surgical history, no medications, and no allergies, and has received her 2-month-old immunizations. She lives with her brother, her biological father, and his girlfriend. Her development is appropriate for age; she tracks, smiles, and is not yet rolling. Vitals were normal, and on physical exam the patient is well appearing and playful, with mild nasal congestion, but good capillary refill and clear lungs. You notice a bruise on her forehead, her father says she fell out of her crib and hit the rails on the side. Her neurological exam is nonfocal.

What do you do now?

DIAGNOSIS

Viral syndromes are common chief complaints in children in the acute care setting with the majority of patients discharged home with anticipatory guidance. However, care must be taken to perform a thorough physical exam, especially in young, nonmobile infants. The infant in this case is not yet mobile, as defined by not yet cruising, which is walking holding on to objects such as furniture. Therefore, in this scenario, the presence of a bruise on physical exam should raise concern for nonaccidental trauma.

Cutaneous injuries such as bruises, burns, bite marks, lacerations, abrasions, and petechiae are skin injuries that are not only the most common accidental injuries but also the most common form of physical child abuse. About 50% to 60% of all physical abuse cases have skin injuries, with or without other injuries.[1]

Cutaneous injuries may fall under the category of sentinel injuries, which are minor inflicted injuries that can go unrecognized by physicians as a manifestation of nonaccidental trauma, and occur prior to the child being recognized as the victim of physical abuse. Cutaneous injuries are usually identified in 25% of abused infants and in one-third of those with abusive head trauma.[2] Jenny et al. found that 20 out of 54 missed abusive head traumas had some facial or head bruising that was not related to presenting symptoms.[3]

BRUISES

Bruises must be considered in the context of a child's age and development. Bruises are uncommon in children less than 6 months of age, as children in this age group are considered precruisers and thus not mobile. Accidental injuries are more common as the patient becomes increasingly more mobile (crawling, pulling to stand, and walking, respectively). Wedgewood et al. demonstrated that 24% of infants who were cruising had a bruise, but no bruises were found in infants not yet cruising. Sugar et al. showed that only 2.2% of precruisers had bruises when compared to 17.8% of cruisers and 51.9% of ambulatory toddlers. These statistics lead to the understanding that "If the infant is not cruising, they should not be bruising."[4]

Knowledge of the child's age and stage of development will also put into the context the location of the bruise (Table 15.1). Injuries to the head and face are more common in children ages 10 to 18 months but less common in children older than 4 years. Children older than 4 have much better control over their motor skills and are more likely to protect their head during a fall.[1] Bruises on the lower legs are more common in children over 18 months of age.

The TEN4 FACES mnemonic is helpful in considering injury and risk. It notes the following patterns should raise concern for child physical abuse:

- Bruising to the **torso, ear, neck** for children under 4 years of age.
- Any bruising in children **under 4 months** of age.
- Any injuries of the frenulum, auricular area, cheeks, eyelids, and sclera.[2]

The TEN4 bruising clinical prediction rule had a sensitivity of 97% and specificity of 87% for predicting abuse, and 72% of abusive head trauma patients had TEN4 bruising.[5]

TABLE 15.1. **Injury Locations[6] in Context with History and Age**

Accidental Injury Locations	Inflicted Injury Locations
Shins	Upper arms
Lower arms	Upper anterior and medial thighs
Under chin	Trunk
Forehead	Genitalia
Hips	Buttocks
Elbows	Face
Ankles	Ears
	Neck
	Soles of feet
	Frenulum
	Auricular area
	Cheeks
	Eyelids
	Sclera
	Head

Source: Kellogg ND. Evaluation of Suspected Child Physical Abuse. *Pediatrics.* 2007;119(6):1232–41.

Bruises tend to be more common in walking children, they tend to be small and over bony prominences, usually extensor surfaces and on the front of the body. Injuries that are more likely to be abusive occur away from the bony prominences, are larger, multiple, and may involve the head, neck, face, medial thighs, buttocks, trunk, arm, and soles of feet.[6]

Patterned injuries are concerning regardless of the age of the patient and reflect the object that struck the child or the child impacted, such as a hand, belt, shoes, or ropes.[1] Flexible objects such as belts have the ability to contour around a curve, such as from the front of the abdomen to the back when it is swung, versus inflexible objects that do not contour.

Other injuries seen in nonaccidental trauma include subgaleal hematomas, bite marks, petechiae of face and neck, purpura of the external ear, and subungual hematomas. Subgaleal hematomas may occur with violent pulling of a child's hair. Bite marks are patterned injuries generally in an ovoid pattern and have central ecchymosis.[2] An adult human bite may be differentiated from a child's bite by an intercanine distance of more than 2 cm.[6] Bite marks in specific can be used to get forensic information if swabbed with sterile water.[2] Facial and neck petechiae occur from attempted strangulation or suffocation. Purpura of the external ear may occur secondary to a blow to the side of the head or pulling or pinching the ear. Other concerning injuries include bruises to the gluteal cleft from a blow to the buttocks and subungual hematomas from biting child's finger or hitting the fingers.[1]

Documentation of bruises involves taking clear images with measurement and detailed descriptions in the medical records about location, size, and shape. Ensure that you place the patient's name, medical record number, date of birth, and date of exam to appropriately identify the photo. Use a neutral background with good lighting. Take images from different angles and distances and include landmarks to better understand the location. Use the rule of 3, which states to take 2 shots of 3 orientations: full body, medium, and close up, and include a color wheel or a scale to give a better idea to the viewers of the injury.[7]

It is important to note that the color of a bruise can be described, however; the color of a bruise does not accurately correlate with the age of a bruise. Maguire et al. described how the accuracy of aging a bruise within 24 hours of its occurrence was less than 50%, mostly because any color can be present at any time and the human eye is not accurate at discriminating these colors.[8]

Medical evaluation of bruises, especially in young infants, should consider bleeding disorders such as von Willebrand disease, hemophilia, immune thrombocytopenia purpura, and vitamin K deficiency in the differential. Ask specific questions about whether or not there was prolonged bleeding during interventions such as vaccines, circumcision, sutures, or dental procedures and about medication use such as NSAID that could alter platelet function. Note if the child has had prior episodes of bruising, joint swelling, hematuria, melena, gingival bleeding, and nosebleeds. In pubertal females ask about menses history and if there is any menorrhagia.[9] Family history is also important and should include queries regarding bleeding issues in the family and any females with menorrhagia.

The initial evaluation should include a complete blood count (CBC) (look for thrombocytopenia or anemia), prothrombin time/activated partial thromboplastin time (PT/aPTT). Abnormalities in the screening laboratory evaluation may require a consult to hematology for more extensive evaluation, which may include mixing studies, von Willebrand antigen, Factor VIII activity, Factor IX activity, ristocentin cofactor, PFA-100, and platelet aggregation studies.[9]

Since bruising may be an external manifestation of more extensive internal injury, including abdominal trauma, extremity fractures, or head trauma, further investigation is necessary in order to reveal these more significant injuries. The skeletal survey is mandatory in all cases of suspected physical abuse in children younger than 2 years of age. Skeletal surveys have been shown, in 10%–30% of cases, to reveal occult fractures and facilitate diagnosis and treatment of a child with suspected nonaccidental injuries. Expert consensus recommends in infants less than 6 months of age a skeletal survey should be performed for all bruises except for an infant with a history of a fall and bruises in the T-shaped zone (forehead, upper lip and chin), frontal scalp, or extremity bony prominences.[10] For infants 6–9 months of age a skeletal survey was recommended for multiple bruises, or any bruising in cheek/eye area, upper arm, upper leg, ear, neck, or torso. In infants 9–12 months of age a skeletal survey was recommended for bruising of the cheek/eye area, upper arm, upper leg, ear, neck, torso, hand, or foot.[10]

Neuroimaging should be considered for any child less than 2 years of age with injuries suspicious for nonaccidental injury. Inflicted head trauma is frequently undetected, in a review of hospitalized children with abusive head trauma 31% cases were missed, with an average of 2.8 physician visits prior to recognition.[11] Screening for occult abdominal trauma should also be considered. Elevation of liver function tests above 80 IU/L for AST or ALT require additional imaging (CT scan of the abdomen with contrast).[6,12] Ophthalmology exam should be performed when there are any neurological symptoms or findings on CT of the head.[2]

BURNS

Burns are another type of cutaneous injury, which can be caused by many different methods such as thermal, electrical, chemical, or radiation.[1] Thermal burns are the most common type of abusive injury and include both scald and contact burns as the most common subgroups. The most well-known type of inflicted burn is forced immersion scald burns, where part of the child is forcibly placed into prolonged contact with hot water, usually the tub. In contrast to accidental burn injuries, immersion scald burns have a clear demarcation, an absence of splash marks, clear tide levels and generally involve the lower trunk, buttocks, perineum, arms, and legs and appear as "stocking or glove" burns at the feet and hands. Flexor surfaces are usually spared.[1,13] While forced immersion burns are highly concerning for child physical abuse, not all immersion burns are inflicted. Care must be taken to elicit a clear history in the context of a patient's development. Accidental scald burns due to spill injuries tend to be irregular, asymmetrical, and rarely full thickness burns. They usually happen from children pulling liquid onto themselves that can land on the anterior face, head, neck, palmar surfaces of hand, arms, or anterior shoulder and chest.[1] It is important to consider developmental ability in the context of the clinical history.

Patterned contact burns may include cigarette burns that cause a circular, uniform-sized deep burn typically found on hands and feet.[1] It is important to remember that not all circular burns are from cigarettes, and again a differential diagnosis must be considered. Iron burns are linear or triangular in pattern.[1] With contact burns, the consideration in the appearance of movement is important. Injuries with irregular borders may suggest movement and therefore may be less likely to be inflicted. However, even when child physical abuse is excluded, consideration must be given to the possibility that the injury was a result of neglectful behavior. Additionally, when there is a delay to care, concerns should be raised for medical neglect as well in the context of the patient's clinical presentation.[13]

It is also important to recognize that patterned marks may be the result of cultural practices such as cupping or coining. Cupping involves placement of a small, heated jar that causes a darkish blue circular bruise, and is used in some cultures to suck out illnesses. Coining causes a long wide mark or oval irregular bordered bruise.[7]

CASE CONCLUSION

The patient has a 5-year-old brother, and therefore concerns should be raised for all siblings where nonaccidental trauma is suspected. Verbal children may be helpful in providing corroborating information if they may have witnessed an abusive or accidental event resulting in an injury. Furthermore, the physician must also consider whether there is a need for medical intervention for siblings. Specifically, the literature suggests that twins and siblings less than 2 years of age require specific medical evaluation. Siblings greater than 2 years of age may require a thorough physical exam and further information gathering. If siblings are less than 2 years, a skeletal survey should be performed even if there are no signs on a physical exam.[14]

Anywhere during this process, if the concern is there for child abuse, child protective services should be involved. All 50 states have mandated reporting that does not require proof before reporting, just suspicion. The family should be made aware of the reporting and that it is mandatory and necessary when patients in this age come with these concerns and is part of routine care. Documentation must be done thoroughly in these cases because many services such as law enforcement, child protective services, and the court system may refer to them.[6]

In the particular case discussed in this chapter, the patient had a CT head scan done, which showed bilateral small to moderate subdural hematomas in multiple stages. Ophthalmology was consulted and noted bilateral retinal hemorrhages with different stages of healing. Skeletal survey and liver enzymes done were normal. Patient was in the hospital until child protective services were able to place her in foster care. The sibling physical exam was unremarkable and thus he was not taken into custody of child protective services.

KEY POINTS TO REMEMBER

· Typical accidental bruise locations in mobile children: Shins, lower arms, under chin, forehead, hips, elbows, ankles.[6]
· Typical inflicted bruises locations: Upper arms, upper anterior thighs, trunk, genitalia, buttocks, face, ears, neck.[6]
· TEN4 rule: bruising of Torso, Ear, Neck in children <4 years old or any bruising in children <4 months of age should raise concern.[2]
· You cannot date an injury based on the color of a bruise.[8]
· CBC, PT, and aPTT are good initial tests to rule out possible bleeding disorders.[9]
· Accidental scald burns tend to be irregular, asymmetrical, and rarely full thickness burns. Immersion burns have clear demarcation and an absence of splash marks and clear tide levels.[1]

Further Reading

1. Jenny C, Reece R. Cutaneous manifestations of child abuse. In: B Diane, ed. *Child Abuse Medical Diagnosis and Management.* 3rd ed. American Academy of Pediatrics; 2009:19–53.
2. Christian CW, Committee on Child Abuse and Neglect AeAoP. The evaluation of suspected child physical abuse. *Pediatrics.* 2015;135(5):e1337–54.
3. Jenny C, Hymel KP, Ritzen A, Reinert SE, Hay TC. Analysis of missed cases of abusive head trauma. *JAMA.* 1999;281(7):621–6.
4. Sugar NF, Taylor JA, Feldman KW. Bruises in infants and toddlers: those who don't cruise rarely bruise. Puget Sound Pediatric Research Network. *Arch Pediatr Adolesc Med.* 1999;153(4):399–403.
5. Tiyyagura GB, Beucher M. Bechtel, K. Nonaccidental injury in pediatric patients: detection, evaluation, and treatment. *Pediatr Emerg Med Pract.* 2017;14:1–32.
6. Kellogg ND. Evaluation of suspected child physical abuse. *Pediatrics.* 2007;119(6):1232–41.

7. Botash A. Child abuse evaluation & treatment for medical providers. http://www.childabusemd.com/. Published 2005. Accessed May 24, 2019.

8. Maguire S, Mann MK, Sibert J, Kemp A. Can you age bruises accurately in children? a systematic review. *Arch Dis Child.* 2005;90(2):187–9.

9. Savage W, Takemoto C. Bleeding and bruising. *Contemp Pediatr.* 2009;26:60–68.

10. Wood JN, French B, Song L, Feudtner C. Evaluation for occult fractures in injured children. *Pediatrics.* 2015;136(2):232–40.

11. Ward MG, King WJ, Bennett S. From bruises to brain injury: the physician's role in the assessment of inflicted traumatic head injury. *Paediatr Child Health.* 2013;18(8):423–4.

12. Lindberg DM, Shapiro RA, Blood EA, Steiner RD, Berger RP. Utility of hepatic transaminases in children with concern for abuse. *Pediatrics.* 2013;131(2):268–75.

13. Andronicus M, Oates RK, Peat J, Spalding S, Martin H. Non-accidental burns in children. *Burns.* 1998;24:552–8.

14. Lindberg DM, Shapiro RA, Laskey AL, et al. Prevalence of abusive injuries in siblings and household contacts of physically abused children. *Pediatrics.* 2012;130(2):193–201.

16 Who's Doing the Twist?

Shilpa Hari, Dana Kaplan, and
Isabel A. Barata

A 5-month-old male presents to the ED with his mother for "not moving his right arm." Mom says he was sleeping in his crib when she heard him "shriek." When she went to check on him, he was laying on top of his right arm. He was born full-term via vaginal delivery with no noted birth trauma. He has no past medical history or surgical history, is on no medications, and has no allergies and his immunizations are up to date. He lives with his 2-year-old brother and his mother. His development is within normal limits for age, and he can roll but is not yet crawling or cruising. Vitals are normal and on physical exam patient is holding his right arm to the side, not moving it and cries when it is manipulated, there is no obvious deformity or clavicular tenderness. Radiograph demonstrates a spiral humerus fracture of the right arm that is slightly displaced.

What do you do now?

DIAGNOSIS

In this case of a spiral humerus fracture of the right arm, the next step should be to consider possible etiologies of the fracture, other associated injuries and diagnostic studies and consults that are necessary.

In determining the cause, the most important aspect is to see if the clinical history is consistent with the injury. Age and development are paramount in weighing this consideration. In general, at 4 months of age, an infant can roll from their stomach to their back and at roughly 6 months of age, the infant can roll from their back to their stomach.[1] In general, children less than 9 months are considered precruisers and thus not mobile, accidental injuries due to pulling to stand and walking are less likely in this age group. However, while these are the averages, children may develop earlier, and therefore objective information to confirm their developmental level is helpful. For example, if a parent states their 7-month-old is cruising, one can ask to see a video of this behavior or have the patient cruise in the exam room.

Fractures in young children fall under the category of sentinel injuries, which are minor inflicted injuries that can go unrecognized by physicians as a form of physical abuse. These sentinel injuries are usually identified in 25% of abused infants.[2] Approximately 12%–20% of physical abuse cases in infants and toddlers are fractures. Only 2% of accidental fractures are in children under 18 months of age and approximately 80% of abuse fractures occur in the same age group.[3] The first point to consider when evaluating the plausibility of an injury is the history; is this a vague/unclear history, changing history, history that is absent, or a history where the way the injury occurred does not seem plausible in the context of clinical practice and/or the reported literature. In order to evaluate appropriately, detailed questions need to be asked which involve the initial position and final position of the child, when the patient was last clinically well, or the circumstances of the patient (e.g., patient was placed on a pillow and fell) as examples.[2,4,5] Sometimes a scene reenactment is helpful. Determine whether there was a delay in seeking care or whether there was a witness during the episode. Learn about social history, who all lives at home, whether there are siblings that could be playing with the infant, substance abuse, parental stress factors like domestic violence, separation, mental health disorders, or previous child protective services involvement.[2,5] While these factors do not make a diagnosis of abuse, they are important social risk factors to consider. It is also important to inquire about birth history such as prematurity, low birth weight, and birth trauma.[5]

For the physical exam, it is crucial to note a thorough skin exam to look for bruises, lacerations, and abrasions and to photograph any that raise suspicion. In nonmobile infants, look at the frenulum, ears, and skin folds and remember to remove the diaper. It is imperative that the neurological status and head circumference of the baby be noted given that fractures are considered sentinel injuries and seen in one-third of those with abusive head trauma.[2,5]

When concerns for child physical abuse are raised, further medical workup is necessary. In children less than 2 years of age, skeletal surveys are recommended testing for suspected cases of child abuse. It consists of 19 images involving frontal and lateral projections for the skull, spine, chest, and oblique views for the ribs to look for posterior rib fractures and frontal views for the appendicular skeleton. The skull needs 4 views, but a CT 3D model version could also be used.[3,6,7] Fractures may not be visible in the initial skeletal survey, especially rib fractures and classic metaphyseal lesions, thus there should be a follow-up skeletal survey done in 2 weeks, doing so can improve the number of fractures diagnosed by 25%.[2] Rib fractures in particular are usually asymptomatic and frequently missed in imaging because they are not displaced; it is possible to see callus formation 7–10 days after the injury, however, which would be picked up on the repeat skeletal survey. This is true for most of the bones' healing phases and could help with dating a fracture.[6,7]

Other imaging modalities are possible but are usually adjunctive; an example is bone scans, which are used for detecting rib fractures, subperiosteal bone formation, and shaft fractures, but are not good for classic metaphyseal lesions and skull fractures. CT of the chest or MRI could also look for rib fractures but would only be useful if a skeletal survey were not conclusive.[7]

In addition to a skeletal survey, head imaging must be considered. Abusive head trauma is a leading cause of mortality and can occur without any neurological symptoms, thus it can only be found via imaging. A cranial computed tomography (CT) should be considered for children less than 1 year of age with or without neurologic symptoms where abuse is suspected.[2] Specifically children less than 6 months of age with any concerning injury should have head imaging performed as the incidence of abusive head trauma is highest in this age group due to crying peaking around 3 months of age.[8] Ophthalmology exam should be performed when there are any neurological symptoms or findings on a CT of the head.[2]

Inflicted abdominal injury can be missed due to lack of bruising and lack of specific symptoms; however, it is the second leading cause of mortality from physical abuse.[2] It tends to happen to younger patients and is more likely to have a delayed presentation frequently occurring in hollow viscera.[5] Therefore, liver function tests should be evaluated in young patients where child physical abuse is considered. A level of >80 IU/L for AST or ALT is suggestive of trauma that requires more evaluation.[9] A urinalysis could also indicate trauma to the kidneys or urinary tract.[5] Imaging such as a CT of the abdomen should be considered if levels are elevated.[9]

Other diagnostic evaluation to consider in patients with fractures relates to a differential diagnosis for nonaccidental trauma, which includes osteogenesis imperfecta and Vitamin D deficiency rickets. Laboratory evaluation should include serum magnesium, calcium, phosphorus, alkaline phosphatase, 25 hydroxyvitamin D, and parathyroid hormone.[3] For osteogenesis imperfecta, genetic testing is available; however, the results would not be returned during the emergency department evaluation. Instead inquire about symptoms and signs such as macrocephaly, blue sclera, poor dentition, hearing impairment, limb deformities, short stature, and family history including consanguinity.[3] Imaging with normal bone mineralization and structure would make many of these disease entities less likely.

There is a misconception that certain diaphyseal fracture patterns such as spiral, transverse, or oblique are more specific for abuse. Diaphyseal fractures are common accidental and nonaccidental injuries, so in isolation they are not pathognomonic for abuse.[4] However, there are certain fractures that are highly specific for abuse, as seen in Table 16.1, such as classic metaphyseal lesions also known as "bucket handle" or "corner fracture," posterior rib fractures,scapular, spinous process, and sternal fractures.[4,7] Classic metaphyseal lesions (CMLs) usually are due to torsion and traction shearing forces, which occurs when an infant's extremity is twisted or pulled.[3] Rib fractures found posteromedial are more

TABLE 16.1. **Specificity of Fractures**[4]

High Specificity	Moderate Specificity	Low Specificity
Classic Metaphyseal Fractures	Multiple Fractures	Clavicular Fractures
Posterior Rib Fractures	Bilateral Fractures	Long Bone Shaft Fractures
Scapular Fractures	Fractures of Different Ages	Subperiosteal Bone Formation
Spinous Process Fractures	Epiphyseal Separations	Linear Skull Fractures
Sternal Fractures	Vertebral Body Fractures and Subluxations	
	Digital Fractures	
	Complex or Depressed Skull Fractures	

Source: Sink EL, Hyman JE, Matheny T, Georgopoulos G, Kleinman P. Child abuse: the role of the orthopaedic surgeon in nonaccidental trauma. *Clin Orthop Relat Res.* 2011;469(3):790–7.

correlated with abuse and are caused by anterior–posterior compression.[3] Moderately specific injury patterns are multiple fractures, especially if bilateral, fractures of different ages, epiphyseal separations, vertebral body fractures and subluxations, digital fractures, and complex or depressed skull fractures. Low-specificity fractures include clavicular fractures, long-bone shaft fractures, subperiosteal bone formation, and linear skull fractures.[4,7] Fractures should be considered in the context of the history, age, and development. Therefore, a humerus fracture in a nonmobile infant has higher potential for abuse, whereas the same fracture in a mobile toddler may be less specific for abuse.[4]

CASE CONCLUSION

The patient has a 2-year-old brother and based on this injury there is concern for his safety as well. The literature suggests that in twins and siblings less than 2 years of age, a skeletal survey should be performed even if there are no signs of injury on a physical exam. Children older than 2 years of age should have a thorough physical exam and appropriate information gathering when the patient is verbal.[10]

Anywhere during this process, if the concern is there for child abuse, child protective services should be involved. All 50 states have mandated reporting that does not require proof before reporting, just suspicion. The family should be made aware of the reporting and that it is mandatory and necessary when patients in this age come with these concerns and is part of routine care. Documentation must be done thoroughly in these cases because many services such as law enforcement, child protective services, and the court system may refer to them.[5]

In this particular case, a skeletal survey done showed no other fractures, and the orthopedic team consulted recommended no immobilization and outpatient follow-up. Laboratory workup looking for differential diagnoses such as rickets was negative. CT head performed was also negative. Child protective services were involved and placed the patient in foster care. The 2-year-old brother had a physical exam and skeletal survey that was unremarkable, and he stayed with the mother.

KEY POINTS TO REMEMBER

- Highly specific fractures for abuse are: CML, posterior rib, scapular, spinous process, and sternal fractures.[7]
- Any child under 2 years of age needs a skeletal survey if you are concerned for abuse, and a repeat skeletal survey in 2 weeks' time.[2]
- Twins and siblings less than 2 years of age should get a skeletal survey as well, if injury is severe in initial case patient.[10]
- Lab work: serum magnesium, calcium, phosphorus, alkaline phosphatase, 25 hydroxyvitamin D, parathyroid hormone.[3]
- CT of the head should be performed even if the infant does not have any neurologic findings, especially for children less than 1 year of age.[2]
- Liver function tests with a level of >80 IU/L for AST or ALT are suggestive of abdominal trauma and require further evaluation.[9]

Further Reading

1. *Bright Futures: Guidelines for Health Supervision of Infants, Children, and Adolescents.* 3rd ed. Elk Grove Village, IL: American Academy of Pediatrics; 2008.
2. Christian CW. Committee on Child Abuse and Neglect AeAoP. The evaluation of suspected child physical abuse. *Pediatrics.* 2015;135(5):e1337–54.
3. Flaherty EG, Perez-Rossello JM, Levine MA, et al. Evaluating children with fractures for child physical abuse. *Pediatrics.* 2014;133(2):e477–89.
4. Sink EL, Hyman JE, Matheny T, Georgopoulos G, Kleinman P. Child abuse: the role of the orthopaedic surgeon in nonaccidental trauma. *Clin Orthop Relat Res.* 2011;469(3):790–7.
5. Kellogg ND. Evaluation of suspected child physical abuse. *Pediatrics.* 2007;119(6):1232–41.
6. Cooperman DR, Merten DF. Skeletal manifestations of child abuse. In: D Beausoleil, ed. *Child Abuse Medical Diagnosis and Management.* 3rd ed. American Academy of Pediatrics; 2009:121–67.
7. Botash A. Child Abuse Evaluation and Treatment for Medical Providers. http://www.childabusemd.com/. Published 2005. Accessed May 24, 2019.
8. Hernandez BS. Child Abuse (Non-Accidental Trauma). https://www.saem.org/cdem/education/online-education/peds-em-curriculum/gu-ob/child-abuse-(non-accidental-trauma). Published 2019. Accessed June 6, 2019.
9. Lindberg DM, Shapiro RA, Blood EA, Steiner RD, Berger RP. Utility of hepatic transaminases in children with concern for abuse. *Pediatrics.* 2013;131(2):268–75.
10. Lindberg DM, Shapiro RA, Laskey AL, et al. Prevalence of abusive injuries in siblings and household contacts of physically abused children. *Pediatrics.* 2012;130(2):193–201.

17 It's "Nap" Time!

Angela Hua

A 3-year-old boy is brought in by his mother, crying and refusing to bear weight on his right foot. Just prior to arrival in the emergency department, he had accidentally knocked a drinking glass off the coffee table. Startled, he jumped and stepped onto broken glass fragments. On cursory examination, he has three small lacerations on the bottom of his right foot. An x-ray obtained shows two small glass fragments embedded in the foot. However, the patient is refusing any attempt at close examination. Whenever he is approached, he starts to cry harder, kicking and twisting away, despite his mother's best efforts to hold his foot still.

What do you do now?

DISCUSSION

In the case of this 3-year-old boy, it is clear that he has lacerations on his foot causing pain, and the emergency physician should be mindful of addressing pediatric pain. In addition to pain, there is a significant component of anxiety that contributes to this child's unwillingness to be closely examined. However, careful examination is paramount for foreign body removal as well as laceration repair. In the approach to a child, first, attempt to establish a rapport with the patient. Speak in language that resonates with the child, and try to reassure the child. Provide distraction, using videos, books, music, toys, and so forth. Parents and child life specialists can be of great assistance in trying to calm and distract the pediatric patient. Administer pain medications, such as acetaminophen (15 mg/kg) and/or ibuprofen (10 mg/kg). Apply LET (lidocaine/epi/tetracaine) to the lacerations for analgesia, if the child will allow someone to touch the area. If the child continues to be too anxious to cooperate with exploring the wound for foreign body removal, the next step would be to consider sedation.

As set forth by the American Academy of Pediatrics,

> The goals of sedation in the pediatric patient for diagnostic and therapeutic procedures are as follows: (1) to guard the patient's safety and welfare; (2) to minimize physical discomfort and pain; (3) to control anxiety, minimize psychological trauma, and maximize the potential for amnesia; (4) to modify behavior and/or movement so as to allow the safe completion of the procedure; and (5) to return the patient to a state in which discharge from medical/dental supervision is safe, as determined by recognized criteria.[1]

DEFINITIONS OF SEDATION

There are multiple levels of sedation to consider. For most procedural sedations in the emergency department, the patient is brought to a mild, moderate, or deep sedation. Below are the definitions from the American Society of Anesthesiologists:

Minimal sedation: Near-baseline level of alertness; patients respond normally to verbal commands; ventilatory and cardiovascular functions are unaffected; commonly used to facilitate minor procedures.[2]

Moderate sedation: Pharmacologically induced depression of consciousness; patients respond purposefully to verbal commands, with or without light tactile stimulation; ventilatory and cardiovascular functions preserved.[2]

Deep sedation: Depression of consciousness; patients not easily aroused but respond purposefully after repeated or painful stimulation; may have impaired ability to maintain ventilatory function; cardiovascular function usually maintained.[2]

General anesthesia: Sedation in which patient is unresponsive to all stimuli; impaired ventilatory function, loss of airway protective reflexes; patients often require assistance in maintaining airway; cardiovascular function may be impaired.[2]

CANDIDACY FOR SEDATION

Prior to undertaking a sedation, it is necessary to perform an assessment of whether the patient is an appropriate candidate for sedation. Obtain an "AMPLE" history: allergies, medications, past history, last meal, and other events; inquire about any previous anesthesia history. Perform a thorough physical exam, including airway assessment. Evaluate the patient's sedation risk using a classification system developed by the American Society of Anesthesiology (ASA). ASA 1 and 2 are considered low-risk sedation patient populations; ASA 3 and 4 are high-risk populations.[3] Please refer to Table 17.1 for the ASA class score.

As for the topic of last meal/oral intake, the current ASA recommendations for fasting before elective procedures are as follows: clear liquids—2 hours; breast milk—4 hours; other milk and solids—6 hours.[4] However, two large prospective studies of procedural sedation involving ketamine, versed, and fentanyl showed no difference in complications between patients who met fasting guidelines versus those who did not.[5,6] According to the 2008 clinical policy set out by the American College of Emergency Physicians (ACEP), in answer to the critical question, "Should pediatric patients undergo a

TABLE 17.1. **ASA Classification**[3]

Classification	Definition
ASA I	A normal healthy patient
ASA II	A patient with mild systemic disease
ASA III	A patient with severe systemic disease
ASA IV	A patient with severe systemic disease that is a constant threat to life
ASA V	A moribund patient who is not expected to survive without an operation
ASA VI	A declared brain-dead patient whose organs are being removed for donor purposes

period of preprocedural fasting to decrease the incidence of clinically important complications during procedural sedation in the ED?," the level B recommendation is that "procedural sedation may be safely administered to pediatric patients in the ED who have had recent oral intake."[7]

MONITORING DURING SEDATION

During the sedation, it is important to closely monitor the blood pressure, heart rate, respiratory rate, use continuous pulse oximetry, and document these numbers every 5 minutes. Additionally, continuous capnography is quite a useful monitoring tool. Capnography detects hypoventilation, which may occur prior to desaturation. It is particularly helpful if the provider is also using supplemental oxygen during the sedation. The American Academy of Pediatrics (AAP) guidelines of 2016 specifically notes that "monitoring of ventilation by 1) capnography (preferred) or 2) amplified, audible pretracheal stethoscope or precordial stethoscope is strongly recommended."[8]

Keep in mind that children are not simply small adults. Pediatric patients are more likely to have airway obstruction during sedation secondary to a relatively larger tongue, epiglottis, and occiput. Additionally, children's oxygen levels desaturate more rapidly after apnea as compared to even moderately ill adults. Finally, children require more frequent sedation dosing, and their sedation level may often be more difficult to assess. It is imperative that drug dosages be calculated based on actual weight measured that day, not an estimate given by a parent. Often, despite careful calculations, children may become more deeply sedated than intended. Ensure that size and age appropriate resuscitation equipment are at beside.

SEDATION AGENTS

There are numerous agents that may be used for sedation, each with their pros and cons. Consider the duration of procedure, drug characteristics and side effect profile, and familiarity of staff with the agent. See Table 17.2 for a list of medications and their properties.

Midazolam
Midazolam is one of the most commonly used benzodiazepines. It is a short-acting, water-soluble drug that acts by binding with GABA receptors. It has a good safety record, and provides potent sedation, anxiolysis, and amnesia. It would be a great choice in short procedures such as this foreign body case, thanks to its rapid onset and short duration. Keep in mind that it has no analgesic effect.

Barbiturates
Barbiturates act on the central nervous system and can rapidly induce sedation. Pentobarbital is often used for radiologic procedures, such as CT/MRI scans, that require children to be still. Propofol has a rapid onset of action and rapid recovery time, which is quite useful for many emergency department procedures requiring sedation. The effects of propofol on mental status are dose-dependent, and can range from light sedation to general anesthesia. It may cause decreased cardiac output and severe hypotension, as well as profound respiratory depression and apnea. Close monitoring is imperative. Propofol is contraindicated in patients with egg or soybean allergy.

Narcotics
Fentanyl and morphine are common choices, and both help with pain management. Fentanyl is preferred because of its rapid onset of action, rapid elimination, and lack of histamine release.

TABLE 17.2. **Sedation Medications**

Medication	Dose	Onset of Action	Duration Of action	Special Considerations
Midazolam	PO 0.5–0.75mg/ kg IN/SL 0.2–0.5mg/kg IV 0.05–0.1mg/ kg	PO 15–20 min IN/SL 10–15 min IV 1–3 min	PO 60–90 min IN/SL 60 min IV 10–30 min	Short acting, good safety record, provides potent sedation, anxiolysis, and amnesia. Contraindicated with shock and narrow angle glaucoma. May be reversed with flumazenil (0.01 mg/kg IV)
Pentobarbital	IM 2–6 mg/kg IV 1–3 mg/kg	IM 10–15 min IV 1 min	IM 1–4 hr IV min	Often used for radiological procedures that require children to be still (i.e., CT/MRI) Beware effects of myocardial depression, hypotension, respiratory depression, bronchospasm
Propofol	IV 1–2 mg/kg, may redose 0.5mg/kg every 2–5 min as needed	30 seconds	10 min	Effects dose-dependent, ranging from light sedation to general anesthesia. Rapid onset and offset, good for short procedures. Beware decreased cardiac output, hypotension, respiratory depression and apnea. Contraindicated in patients with egg or soybean allergy
Fentanyl	IV 1–2 mcg/ kg over 3–5 min, titrate to effect every 3–5 min	1–2 min, with peak effect at 10 min	30–60 min	Rapid onset of action, rapid elimination. Beware that rapid IV administration may cause chest wall rigidity and apnea. May use in combo with benzodiazepine to provide amnesia and analgesia.

Drug	Dose	Onset	Duration	Comments
Morphine	IV 0.1–0.2 mg/kg	5–10 min	2–4 hr	Good agent for procedures with expected longer duration (>30 min). Beware respiratory depression, may reverse effects with Narcan.
Ketamine	IV 1–2 mg/kg IM 2–10 mg/kg	Onset in seconds	10–20 min for sedation 40–45 min for analgesia	Provides analgesia and sedation, rapid onset. Maintains hemodynamic stability, preserves respiratory drive and airway protective reflexes. Complications include laryngospasm, hypersalivation, vomiting, agitation, hallucination, emergence reactions, hypertension, increased intracranial and intraocular pressures. Contraindications: children <3 mo, acute pulmonary infection/disease, tracheal surgery/stenosis, intracranial hypertension, glaucoma or acute globe injury IM ketamine associated with higher rates of adverse events compared to IV.
Etomidate	IV 0.2–0.5 mg/kg Standard induction dose 0.3 mg/kg, may redose 0.1 mg/kg every 5–10min	Onset < 1 min	5–10 min	Induces CNS hypnosis, ultra-short-acting. Rapid IV induction, minimal hemodynamic instability, minimal respiratory depression. Contraindicated in patients with seizure disorder and children <2 yr. Side effects include nausea/vomiting and myoclonic movements. Consider pretreating with fentanyl 1–2 mcg/kg to reduce myoclonus.
Nitrous oxide	50% nitrous oxide delivered via nebulizer in oxygen	3–5 min	Recovery 3–5 min	Analgesic and anxiolytic effects. Titratable to depth of sedation, rapid recovery rate.

Fentanyl is often used in conjunction with a benzodiazepine to provide both amnesia and analgesia. However, if using as a combination, be wary of respiratory depression: dosage should be reduced. Be mindful that respiratory depression may last longer than the period of analgesia. Morphine is the better choice for procedures expected to have longer duration (>30 min). Opiate effects may be reversed with Narcan.

Ketamine

Ketamine is an incredibly useful agent for procedural sedation in the emergency department, providing both analgesia and sedation. It maintains hemodynamic stability and preserves respiratory drive as well as airway protective reflexes. Ketamine has the added benefit of being helpful in patients with reactive airway disease, as it also has bronchodilatory effects. Intramuscular (IM) ketamine seems to be associated with higher respiratory events, higher rates of emesis, and longer recovery period, as compared to IV ketamine. Contraindications include children < 3 months old, acute pulmonary disease or infection, tracheal surgery or stenosis, intracranial hypertension, cardiovascular disease, glaucoma or acute globe injury, psychiatric illness, and a full meal within 3 hours.

Etomidate

Etomidate induces CNS hypnosis, and is ultra-short-acting. It is used for both procedural sedation and induction for rapid sequence intubation. Benefits include rapid IV induction, minimal hemodynamic instability, and minimal respiratory depression. Side effects include nausea/vomiting, and myoclonic movements. It may stimulate seizure activity and inhibit steroid synthesis. It is contraindicated in patients with a seizure disorder and in children younger than 2 years old. Consider pretreating with fentanyl 1–2 mcg/kg to reduce myoclonus. Keep in mind that it does not provide analgesia.

Nitrous Oxide

Nitrous oxide is a gas with both analgesic and anxiolytic effects. It is easily titratable to depth of analgesia and sedation, and also has a rapid recovery time. It is particularly well suited for patients who require more anxiolysis than pain control. It is delivered via nebulizer in oxygen, thus having the added benefit of being needleless. Usually 50% nitrous oxide is delivered as a baseline dose; some machines allow for adjustment of the percentage as patient is inhaling to titrate to desired depth of sedation. Benzodiazepines or opiates may be added for deeper sedation.

AFTER THE PROCEDURE

After receiving sedation, the child should be monitored carefully in an area equipped with the capacity to resuscitate. There should be available suction, oxygen delivery system, and age- and size-appropriate equipment necessary for airway rescue. Vital signs should be recorded every 10–15 minutes. Prior to discharge, there should be appropriate vitals for age. The child should demonstrate appropriate activity for age, and should be easily responsive to verbal stimuli. Oxygen saturation should be at the child's normal base-line. One proposed, easy method of checking sedation effects is to watch the child in a quiet environment to see whether they will spontaneously maintain wakefulness for 20 minutes.[8] If a reversal agent was required, the patient should be observed an additional period of time, as the duration of the sedation drug effects may exceed the duration of the reversal agent (e.g., opiates and naloxone).

CASE CONCLUSION

In this particular case, the 3-year-old boy was persistently too anxious for the emergency physician to safely approach for foreign body removal and laceration repair. A child life specialist and the boy's mother helped distract him and kept him calm while nurses placed an IV in his hand (after placement of a topical agent to numb the area). Ketamine was the agent of choice, as it provides both analgesia and sedation and patients maintain respiratory drive. The two wounds on his foot were then probed, the glass shards were successfully removed with pick-ups, and all three lacerations were closed with simple sutures. The patient returned to his baseline mental status shortly after the ketamine administration, and was documented to have age appropriate vital signs and activity. He was soon discharged, happily walking on both of his feet.

Further Reading

1. Coté CJ, Wilson S. American Academy of Pediatrics, American Academy of Pediatric Dentistry. Guidelines for monitoring and management of pediatric patients before, during, and after sedation for diagnostic and therapeutic procedures: update 2016. *Pediatrics*. 2016;138(1):e20161212.

2. American Society of Anesthesiologists. Continuum of depth of sedation: definition of general anesthesia and levels of sedation/ analgesia. October 21, 2009. Available at: http://www.asahq.org/Home/For-Members/ Clinical-Information/Standards-Guidelines-andStatements.

3. American Society of Anesthesiologists. ASA physical status classification system. October 15, 2014. Available at: https://www.asahq.org/standards-and-guidelines/ asa-physical-status-classification-system.

4. American Society of Anesthesiologist Task Force on Preoperative Fasting. Practice guidelines for operative fasting and the use of pharmacologic agents to reduce the risk of pulmonary aspiration: application to healthy patients undergoing elective procedures: a report by the American Society of Anesthesiologist Task Force on Preoperative Fasting. *Anesthesiology*. 1999; 90:896.

5. Agrawal D, et al. Preprocedural fasting state and adverse events in children undergoing procedural sedation and analgesia in a pediatric emergency department. *Ann Emerg Med*. 2003;42(5):636–46.

6. Roback MG, et al. Preprocedural fasting and adverse events in procedural sedation and analgesia in a pediatric emergency department: are they related? *Ann Emerg Med*. 2004; 44(5):454–9.

7. Mace SE, et al. Clinical policy: critical issues in the sedation of pediatric patients in the emergency department. *Ann Emerg Med*. 2008;51(4):378–99, e1–d57.
8. The Society for Pediatric Sedation. Sedation provider course. 2009. https://www.pedsedation.org/wp-content/uploads/2017/01/SPS_Primer_on_Pediatric_Sedation.pdf. Accessed February 20, 2019.

18 FOOSH—OUCH!

Victor Huang, Nima Jalali, Bryan McCarty, and Philipp J. Underwood

A 12-year-old boy is brought in with right arm pain and an obvious deformity after a fall 1 hour ago. His vital signs are a heart rate of 115 bpm, blood pressure of 110/70 mmHg, respiratory rate of 24 breaths per minute, oxygen saturation of 99% on room air, temperature of 37°C, and weight 40 kg. He says he was running when he tripped forward, bracing the fall with his hands. He reports pain to his right wrist and denies any other areas of pain or injury. He has asthma and uses his albuterol inhaler as needed. He takes no other medications, has no allergies, and has not had any fractures or surgeries in the past.

The physical exam shows moderate swelling, tenderness, and deformity over the dorsal aspect of the right distal forearm with intact skin and a palpable bony step-off. Right elbow and shoulder are normal. Distal to the injury, the patient has brisk capillary refill, intact radial pulse, and normal motor and sensory examination to the radial, median, and ulnar nerve distributions.

What do you do now?

DISCUSSION

This child is presenting with wrist pain and deformity after a fall on outstretched hand (FOOSH). The clinical presentation and imaging is consistent with a dorsally displaced distal radius and ulna fracture, as shown in Figure 18.1.

The initial approach to a traumatic extremity injury should begin with a primary assessment of the patient's airway, breathing, circulation, disability, and exposure. Although orthopedic injuries are often the most prominent, it is important to first assess and treat more critical injuries. During the secondary survey, any orthopedic injuries causing neurovascular compromise should be immediately reduced and immobilized. Extremity injuries not causing neurovascular compromise should be evaluated last after assessing the patient for other traumatic injuries.

The history should include the mechanism of injury, location of pain, presence of additional injuries, and associated complaints of paresthesia, numbness, and weakness. When examining acute traumatic injuries in patients with severe pain, the evaluation should be brief with minimal manipulation in

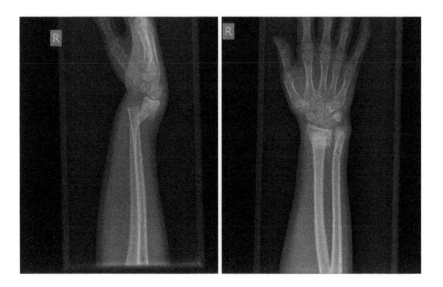

FIGURE 18.1. AP and lateral X-ray of a transverse fracture of the distal radial metaphysis and the ulna with dorsal displacement in a pediatric patient (case courtesy of Dr Sajoscha Sorrentino, Radiopaedia.org, rID: 14840).

order to reduce pain, swelling, and risk of further injury. However, a detailed neurovascular examination distal to the injury should always be completed, including capillary refill, pulse palpation, and motor and sensory examination. After x-rays are performed, a full exam should be done, which includes inspection, palpation, range of motion, and ligament integrity.

The differential diagnosis for FOOSH injury in pediatrics includes Salter-Harris (physeal) fractures, torus (buckle) and greenstick fractures, plastic deformity, and complete fractures of the radius, ulna, and carpal bones including the scaphoid. Other injuries include supracondylar fractures (in a younger age range), wrist and carpal dislocations, fracture-dislocation, carpal instability, distal radioulnar joint (DRUJ) and triangular fibrocartilage complex (TFCC) injuries. It is always important to consider nonaccidental trauma in pediatric trauma, especially when the history is not consistent with the injury or certain patterns of injuries are found.

In the setting of focal pain and tenderness after trauma, plain radiographs are the initial imaging test of choice to assess for fractures and dislocations. The general rule of thumb is to obtain at least 2 orthogonal views of the injured area, and to consider imaging of the joint above and below the injury. Additional views may be obtained based on clinical suspicion. Rarely more advanced imaging is required, including CT (visualize occult fractures) and MRI.

The majority of pediatric fractures (44%) are radius and ulna fractures, which are most commonly seen in children who are 5–14 years old.[1] The most common cause is a fall, typically onto an outstretched hand.

Indications for emergent orthopedic consultation include open fractures, neurovascular compromise, tenting of the skin, and compartment syndrome. Nonemergent orthopedic referral for possible operative repair should be arranged for Salter-Harris type III–V fractures, displaced Salter-Harris H type I and II, and inability to achieve adequate fracture reduction.

Emergent fracture reduction should be performed for fractures with any neurologic or vascular compromise. Displaced fractures should be reduced in the emergency department by a provider who is comfortable with this procedure, often in consultation with an orthopedist.

Analgesia and patient cooperation is a crucial aspect of a successful reduction. Though there are several methods of fracture reduction, a common method is performed in this way: positioning the patient supine on the stretcher, abduct the shoulder to 90 degrees and flex the elbow to 90 degrees. Suspend the hand in the air with a finger trap and hang a weight from the distal humerus for 5–10 minutes to distract the fracture fragments. Then recreate the mechanism of injury and apply longitudinal traction to the distal wrist. Finally, reverse the mechanism of injury to realign the fracture fragments.

Immobilize the fracture with a sugar tong splint with the elbow flexed to 90 degrees, the forearm in neutral position, and the wrist in 10–20 degrees of flexion with 20 degrees of ulnar deviation.

Following any attempts at reduction, a neurovascular examination should be performed and documented. Postreduction radiographs should be obtained to confirm adequate fracture reduction. The patient should be instructed to ice and elevate the fracture, use oral pain medications as needed, and follow-up with the orthopedist in 24–48 hours. They should be given strict return precautions and warning signs to look out for compartment syndrome.

Sedation is often used during fracture reduction to relieve pain and anxiety and to modify behaviors to allow safe completion of a procedure. Occasionally, using parental assistance, distraction, topical anesthetics, cautious preparation, electronic devices, and techniques used by child life specialists can limit the need for pharmacologic sedation. One can also consider performing peripheral nerve blocks, hematoma blocks, or intra-articular blocks to limit the need for sedation as well.

Presedation evaluation involves the assessment of underlying medical problems, which can be quantified with the ASA physical status classification. The patient's airway should be evaluated for aspects that may compromise a patient's respiration such as limited neck mobility, obesity, small mandible, obstructive tonsils, large tongue, or trismus. Equipment should be set up at the bedside in preparation for the procedural sedation, including suction and an oxygen source (Table 18.1). Age- and size-appropriate equipment including oral/nasal airways, bag-valve-masks, supraglottic devices, laryngoscope or glidescope, endotracheal tubes, and rescue devices should be readily available. A patient should be placed on a cardiac monitor with blood pressure, oxygen saturation, and end-tidal carbon dioxide capabilities. Defibrillators with size-appropriate pads should be available.

Preprocedural fasting requirements in urgent sedation situations are controversial. ACEP states that procedural sedation in adults or

TABLE 18.1. **Procedural Sedation Equipment**

Procedural Sedation Checklist

Monitoring: Telemetry, NIBP, Pulse Oximetry, End-Tidal CO_2

Suction

Bag-Valve-Mask connected to an Oxygen Source

Oral and Nasal Airways

Laryngeal Mask Airway with Syringe

Direct and/or Video Laryngoscope and Blades

Endotracheal Tubes (multiple sizes) with Stylets

Adjuncts: Bougie and Difficult Airway Equipment

Defibrillator/AED with Size-appropriate Pads

Medications for Procedural Sedation and Analgesia, Reversal, and Paralytics

pediatrics should not be delayed in the emergency department based on fasting time. Preprocedural fasting has not been shown to reduce the risk of emesis or aspiration when undergoing procedural sedation. However, using agents with less risk of affecting airway reflexes, such as ketamine, may be preferred.

There are many different medications and routes available (Table 18.2). The most commonly used are intranasal versed, and intravenous or

TABLE 18.2. **Common Medications for Conscious Sedation**

Drug	Dose	Duration of Action (Approximate)	Comments/Adverse Effects
Midazolam	.05–0.1 mg/kg IV 0.2–0.6 mg/kg/dose IN	15–30 minutes	Respiratory depression common, especially when used with fentanyl; can be used intranasally for pediatrics
Ketamine	1–2 mg/kg IV	10 minutes	Hypersalivation, emergence phenomenon
Etomidate	0.1–0.15 mg/kg IV	15 minutes	Myoclonic jerks
Propofol	1 mg/kg IV	10 minutes	Hypotension, respiratory depression

intramuscular ketamine. Intranasal medications are useful because they are painless to administer and rapid in onset, and can be used for either sedation or to facilitate IV placement. As with all pediatric procedures, discussion of medications, their potential side effects and procedure details should be discussed with the patient and/or the patient's parents.

After identification of a displaced, dorsally angulated distal radius fracture, our patient underwent successful reduction and splinting after tolerating a hematoma block with 1% lidocaine without epinephrine. He received adjunctive oral acetaminophen and ibuprofen and tolerated the procedure well. He was provided with orthopedic surgery follow-up and strict return precautions including uncontrollable pain, pale or cool fingers, or significant extremity swelling were discussed with the patient and his parents.

KEY POINTS TO REMEMBER

- Use a systematic approach to the initial evaluation of patients with traumatic injuries in order to assess and treat the most critical injuries first.
- Plain radiographs should always include at least two orthogonal views of the injured area, and also should image the joint above and below the injury.
- Emergent orthopedic consultation for open fractures, skin tenting, and compartment syndrome. Fractures with vascular compromise should be reduced immediately.
- Always perform a detailed neurovascular examination before and after any attempt at reduction and immobilization.
- Analgesia with medications and local anesthetics, along with procedural sedation are crucial for successful of the reduction.
- Use a systemic approach to prepare for the sedation, including airway evaluation, monitoring equipment, and back-up airway equipment.

Further Reading

1. Chung KC, Spilson SV. The frequency and epidemiology of hand and forearm fractures in the United States. *J Hand Surg*. 2001;26(5):908–15. 10.1053/jhsu.2001.26322.

2. Rab GT. Chapter 10. Pediatric orthopedic surgery. In: HB Skinner, PJ McMahon, eds. *Current Diagnosis and Treatment in Orthopedics*. 5th ed. New York, NY: McGraw-Hill; 2014. http://accessmedicine.mhmedical.com/content.aspx?bookid=675&sectionid=45451716. Accessed February 5, 2019.

3. Upton SD, Chorley J. Evaluation of wrist pain and injury in children and adolescents. *UpToDate*, 2019. https://www.uptodate.com/contents/evaluation-of-wrist-pain-and-injury-in-children-and-adolescents?search=Evaluation%20of%20wrist%20pain%20and%20injury%20in%20children%20and%20adolescents&source=search_result&selectedTitle=1~79&usage_type=default&display_rank=1. Accessed February 7, 2019.

4. Aziz F, Doty CI. Orthopedic emergencies. In: C Stone, RL Humphries, eds. *Current Diagnosis and Treatment: Emergency Medicine*. 8th ed. New York, NY: McGraw-Hill. http://accessmedicine.mhmedical.com/content.aspx?bookid=2172&sectionid=16506167. Accessed February 12, 2019.

5. Rhodes J, Erickson MA, Tagawa A, Niswander C. Orthopedics. In: WW Hay Jr, MJ Levin, RR Deterding, MJ Abzug, eds. *Current Diagnosis and Treatment: Pediatrics*. 24th ed. New York, NY: McGraw-Hill. http://accessmedicine.mhmedical.com/content.aspx?bookid=2390&sectionid=189081789. Accessed February 5, 2019.

6. Eiff PM, Hatch R. Radius and ulna fractures. In: *Fracture Management for Primary Care*. 3rd ed. Philadelphia, PA: Elsevier Saunders; 2012: 102–17.

7. Coté CJ, Wilson S. American Academy of Pediatrics, American Academy of Pediatric Dentistry. Guidelines for monitoring and management of pediatric patients before, during, and after sedation for diagnostic and therapeutic procedures: update 2016. *Pediatrics*. 2016;138.

8. ASA Physical Status Classification System. *American Society of Anesthesiologists*. October 15, 2014. www.asahq.org/standards-and-guidelines/asa-physical-status-classification-system.

9. Krauss B, Green SM. Procedural sedation and analgesia in children. *Lancet*. 2006;367(9512):766–80.

10. Procedural Sedation and Analgesia in the Emergency Department. *ACEP Clinical Policies. ACEP*, October 2013. www.acep.org/patient-care/clinical-policies/procedural-sedation-and-analgesia/#sm.00015vwc8okzcdvvtlj28qiw6ltwq.

19 I Have an Owie!!!

Evan Feinberg and Melissa A. McGuire

A 7-year-old boy is brought to the emergency department after a trip and fall off his scooter immediately prior to arrival. He was wearing a helmet, and his mother witnessed the fall. She states he lost balance and fell onto his left arm but did not strike his head or lose consciousness. The boy is crying profusely and is cradling his left arm. He has no known allergies, no pertinent past medical history, and no prior surgeries. His heart rate is 118, blood pressure on his right arm is 118/76, respiratory rate is 26 breaths per minute, oxygen saturation is 99% on room air, and temperature is 98.8°F orally after several attempts at redirecting him with child life and using video on his mother's phone. Examination of his left upper extremity is notable for 2+ radial pulse, capillary refill less than 2 seconds, 4/5 grip strength, and a mid-forearm gross deformity with swelling and bruising but intact skin. The remainder of his physical exam is normal.

What do you do now?

DIAGNOSIS

In this previous healthy child presenting with a traumatic fall and probable forearm fracture, there are several aspects to his initial care. Prompt attention to his pain is prudent both to alleviate his suffering and to allow the provider to properly examine him to determine the extent of his injuries. A splint should be placed that immobilizes the joint above and below the fracture. A physical exam, including a neurovascular exam, will need to be performed on the extremity, the neurovascular exam will need to be repeated after splint placement, and radiographs will need to be taken to evaluate for fractures and dislocations.

In this case, x-rays of the left forearm should be obtained after the boy's pain is adequately controlled. The radiographs reveal closed midshaft fractures of the left radius and ulna with significant displacement (Figure 19.1). In certain fractures, as in this case, intravenous access will need to be obtained for procedural sedation to facilitate a closed reduction and splinting at the bedside or in the operating room. All of this will require the

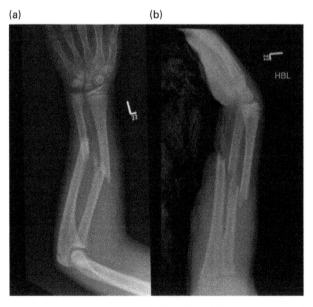

(a)   (b)

FIGURE 19.1. X-rays of the left forearm with AP (a) and lateral (b) views demonstrating midshaft fractures of the radius and ulna with significant angulation.

patient to be calm and cooperative, which he will be unable to do while in significant pain. Appropriate analgesia will also help provide anxiolysis to an understandably frightened and distraught child.

The first priority is to assess a patient's pain so that the provider may then choose the appropriate analgesic method(s) and have a tool to reassess the patient's pain for improvement or worsening. As the pediatric patient population varies significantly in their communicative abilities based on factors including age and developmental stage, a provider must be prepared to assess pain in a different manner than in adult patients, who, in general, are able to convey more recognizable and consistent descriptors for their acute pain.

One such standardized approach to pain assessment is the QUESTT method (Wong et al., 1999) whereby we *Question* the child about their pain, *Use* a pain rating scale, *Evaluate* the child's behavior and physiology including vitals, *Secure* the parent/guardian's involvement, *Take* causes of pain into account, and *Take* action and evaluate results. Commonly used pediatric pain scales include the NIPS (Neonatal/Infant Pain) scale, the FLACC (Faces, Legs, Faces, Activity, Cry, Consolability) scale, the Wong-Baker Faces scale, and the numerical/visual analogue scale.

The NIPS scale (Table 19.1) is used primarily in infants 1 year of age or younger. It uses objective observations of the patient's facial expression, crying, breathing pattern, arm and leg movements, and arousal state. The patient is observed for 1- minute intervals prior to, during, and after an intervention or procedure and each observation period is scored. A score greater than 3 indicates the patient is experiencing pain. The FLACC

TABLE 19.1. **NIPS Neonatal Infant Pain Scale**

NIPS	0 point	1 point	2 points
Facial expression	Relaxed	Contracted	-
Cry	Absent	Mumbling	Vigorous
Breathing	Relaxed	Different than basal	-
Arms	Relaxed	Flexed/stretched	-
Legs	Relaxed	Flexed/stretched	-
Alertness	Sleeping/calm	uncomfortable	-

Maximal score of seven points, considering pain ≥ 3.

scale (Table 19.2) is validated for use in patients from 2 months to 7 years old and is used in patients unable to verbally express their pain. It uses a 0 to 10 scoring system with 0 representing no pain. Each of the five categories (Face, Leg, Arm, Consolability, Cry) receives a score of 0, 1, or 2. The Wong-Baker Faces scale (Figure 19.2) is used in children from approximately 3 to 7 years old who are able to communicate and self-report their pain. This scale uses 6 cartoon faces graded from showing no pain to severe pain in order to aid the patient's self-reporting of pain. The numerical visual analogue scale is used in patients 3 years and older. It involves drawing a line, generally four inches long with the words "no hurt" on

TABLE 19.2. **FLACC (Face, Legs, Activity, Cry, Consolability) Scale**

Behavioral Observation Pain Rating Scale

Categories	Scoring		
	0	1	2
Face	No particular expression or smile; disinterested	Occasional grimace or frown, withdrawn	Frequent to constant frown, clenched jaw, quivering chin
Legs	No position or relaxed	Uneasy, restless, tense	Kicking, or legs drawn up
Activity	Lying quietly, normal position. moves easily	Squirming, shifting back and forth, tense	Arched. rigid, or jerking
Cry	No crying (awake or asleep)	Moans or whimpers, occasional complaint	Crying steadily, screams or sobs, frequent complaints
Consolability	Content, relaxed	Reassured by occasional touching, hugging, or talking to. Distractable	Difficult to console or comfort

Note: Each of the five categories (F) Face; (L) Legs; (A) Activity; (C) Cry; (C) Consolability is scored from 0 to 2, which results in a total score between 0 and 10.

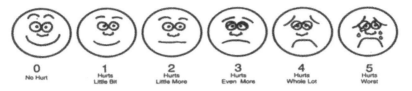

0	1	2	3	4	5
No Hurt	Hurts Little Bit	Hurts Little More	Hurts Even More	Hurts Whole Lot	Hurts Worst

FIGURE 19.2. Wong-Baker Faces scale.

the left and "worst hurt" on the right and the numbers zero through 10 evenly spaced out on the line. The patient is asked to mark where their pain intensity is on the scale. There are variations of this scale, such as using a vertical line fashioned like a thermometer, or incorporating color graded in increasing intensity. In patients 8 years and older, the traditional numerical rating scale is used, similar to that used in adults, by asking them to grade their pain from 0 to 10 with 10 being the worst. It is important to note, however, that age should not be the absolute criteria for choosing a specific scale. Rather, taking into account the child's communicative ability in the moment is essential because it can be influenced by numerous variables including their fears, anxieties, concerns, stress, and so forth.

After assessing the child's pain level, the next decision is to determine analgesic options and the best route of administration. While each clinical setting, whether it be an emergency department, clinic, or office, has its own setup, logistics, and flow, a good practice guideline would be to recognize and appropriately treat patients who are in moderate to severe pain within 20 minutes of arrival and then reevaluate those patients within 60 minutes of their initial pain intervention. This can be accomplished by integrating these goals into the patient workflow on the electronic medical records and triage algorithms/scripts, and by creating an environment where pain is viewed as a "fifth vital sign" and managed as such.

Children should be placed in a position of comfort and spoken to at eye level whenever possible. The fracture should be splinted as soon as possible, immobilizing the joint above and below the site of injury.

Avoid restraining the patient when not required, and distract the patient with modalities such as videos on a family member's electronic device or one provided by the provider's team. Use of child life specialists whenever available can be very valuable while obtaining pharmacologic adjuncts. In patients that are going to require sedation, topical anesthetic cream (such as LMX or EMLA) at least 30–60 minutes prior to anticipated injection/ IV placement, and providing sucrose solution on pacifiers in patients 0 to 12 months of age, will facilitate intravenous access. This child is splinted in triage, mom put his favorite video on her phone, and EMLA is placed on the right arm for future intravenous access.

The least invasive route of medication administration should be used whenever possible, and providers should employ nonpharmacologic strategies regularly in conjunction with pharmacological ones to reduce the amount of medications required. Providers should not avoid using opioids when indicated, but they should use a combination of nonopioid medications in conjunction with opioids whenever possible to help reduce the amount of opioids required. If pain is expected to have a prolonged duration, consider using long-acting formulations and then adding short-acting medication for breakthrough pain as needed. Communication between members of the provider team, the patient, and the parents/guardians is paramount.

There are many options for routes of analgesic administration, including intranasal (IN), oral (PO), rectal (PR), intravenous (IV), and intramuscular (IM). Each route has its own benefits, drawbacks, and logistics. For example, the intranasal route has fast absorption and is relatively noninvasive, but nasal congestion and provider experience can cause variations in the amount of medication successfully delivered. Intramuscular administration can be quicker than IV when IV access has not yet been obtained but is often considered more painful for the patient and will need to be repeated for each subsequent dose.

With regard to analgesic medications, the major categories include acetaminophen, nonsteroidal anti-inflammatories (NSAIDs), opioids, local anesthetics, and dissociatives/sedatives. Each has their own safety and efficacy profiles, contraindications, and scenarios for which they are optimally used. (See Table 19.3.) Additionally, one should not overlook the value of adjuvant therapies such as providing an icepack early on to a musculoskeletal injury or elevating an injured body part.

Acetaminophen and NSAIDs are generally considered first line, for mild to moderate pain. Due to their anti-inflammatory properties, NSAIDs lend

TABLE 19.3. **Pain Medications**

Analgesic	Severity of Pain	Route of Administration	Dose	Mechanism of Action	Special Considerations
NSAIDs	Mild to Moderate (Toradol for certain severe pain)	PO, PR, IV (toradol), IM (toradol)	Ibuprofen 5–10 mg/kg max dose 400 mg Ketorolac IV <2 yrs = 0.25 mg/kg >2 yrs = 0.5 mg/kg max dose 30 mg	Inhibit COX 1 and COX 2 enzymes, reducing prostaglandin production	Do not use in patients under 6 months or under 5–6 kg body weight, if pregnant, or in patients with renal disease or history of severe GI bleed
Acetaminophen	Mild to Moderate	PO, PR, IV	10–15 mg/kg po 4–6 hr	Inhibit prostaglandin production through a yet-to-be-elucidated mechanism in COX pathway	Use with caution in patients with liver disease Acetaminophen does not have anti-inflammatory properties
Opioids	Moderate to Severe	PO, IV, IM, IN (fentanyl)	*Tramadol:* PO 1–2 mg/kg q 4–6 hr; max dose 50–100 mg *Morphine:* IV 0.05–0.1 mg/kg q 2–4 hr or PO 0.15–0.3 mg/kg q 2–4 hr *Hydromorphone:* PO 0.05 mg/kg q 3–4 hr, or IV 15 mcg/kg IV q 2–4 hr, or infusion 2–5 mcg/kg/hr *Oxycodone:* PO 0.1–0.2 mg/kg q 4–6 hr *Fentanyl:* IV 1–2 mcg/kg q 10 min to 1 hr or infusion at 1 mcg/kg/hr	Agonist of endogenous opioid receptors (mu, delta, and kappa). Tramadol also blocks reuptake of serotonin and norepinephrine	Naloxone should be given in the event of an opioid overdose including respiratory depression. Given at 0.1 mcg/kg IV or IM or 2 mg IN Whenever possible, consider coadministering NSAID or acetaminophen when giving an opioid to help reduce the amount of opioid required

(continued)

TABLE 19.3. Continued

Analgesic	Severity of Pain	Route of Administration	Dose	Mechanism of Action	Special Considerations
Ketamine	Moderate to Severe	IV, IM	*Analgesia:* 0.1–0.3 mg/kg IV or 0.5–1 mg/kg IM *Sub-dissociation:* 0.4–0.8 mg/kg IV *Dissociation:* 1–2 mg/kg IV or 2–4 mg/kg IM	NMDA receptor antagonist	If given too quickly or at supratherapeutic doses, may cause respiratory depression, excess salivation, laryngospasm; Emergence phenomenon is possible Controversial risk of ICP elevation
Local Anesthetics	Moderate to Severe	Injection; local or regional block	Lidocaine w/o epi 4.5 mg/kg, max dose 300 mg Lidocaine w/ epi 7 mg/kg, max dose 500	Reversibly inactivates neuron sodium channels; epi, if included, causes local vasoconstriction and increases concentration and duration of anesthetic	Always aspirate before injecting to ensure not in a blood vessel Avoid epi in digits/terminal body parts to avoid risk of necrosis Avoid in areas where compartment syndrome is a concern to avoid increasing volume and pressure

themselves well to musculoskeletal pain and other pain associated with inflammation and swelling.

While it is true there is currently an opioid crisis and this class of medication has habit-forming and addiction potential, opioids are potent, have significant utility in the management of both acute and chronic pain, and should still be considered in the pediatric population when indicated. With that said, care and caution should be exercised when considering prescribing opioids for outpatient use, for example with patients who are being discharged from the hospital after an acute injury such as the patient in this case.

Of note, when considering opioids for analgesia, providers should strongly consider coadministering NSAIDs or acetaminophen or trialing these medications beforehand as they can reduce the need for opioids by 30%–40%. Codeine is a prodrug and should be avoided in pediatric patients, as up to 34% of children are deficient in the codeine metabolizing enzyme CYP2D6, which is expressed in the liver and nervous tissue, and it will therefore not have an analgesic effect on them. Conversely, patients who hypermetabolize codeine can consequently reach dangerous levels of morphine metabolites in their body.

Special mention should be made of administering analgesics intranasally. This route is less invasive and painful than IV and IM administration of medications. Given that children are often already apprehensive about coming to the doctor or hospital, placing an IV in a pediatric patient can be a time- and resource-consuming task, and patients are not always willing or able to take PO medication, the IN route is a useful option to keep in mind and have available. Additionally, assuming the nare is patent (free of blood, significant mucous, etc.), the absorption is rapid and the medication is therefore quick in onset. Of note, the venous plexus of the nose drains in the superior vena cava and bypasses first metabolism by the liver. Volumes of 1 mL can readily be delivered to each nare and multiple doses can also be repeated as needed every 10–15 minutes. Fentanyl in particular is an ideal intranasal medication for moderate to severe pain, as it is concentrated (1–2 mcg/kg per dose), is lipophilic, and has a low molecular weight.

The patient in this case has a fractured left forearm. By administering IN fentanyl to him promptly, the process of obtaining x-rays may be accelerated and placement of a subsequent IV may be better facilitated. Additionally, successfully addressing this patient's pain promptly will foster a better rapport with the child and his parent and reduce provider stress and burnout (related to issues such as compassion fatigue).

Local or regional anesthesia should be considered whenever applicable, as this modality can directly target the source of a patient's pain and mitigate the need for additional medications. Infiltration of local anesthetic also has a very rapid onset. It is a particularly good modality for extremity injuries and for dental pain, especially when used in conjunction with a topical mucous membrane anesthetic such as benzocaine prior to injecting the patient. Ultrasound can greatly facilitate performing certain regional blocks, though provider comfort and experience will also affect the probability of first attempt success. Drawbacks to this method include variable provider experience and comfort, the use of an invasive injection, and potentially limited access and availability to ultrasound and/or sufficiently long and thin needles for infiltration.

Ketamine is a dissociative anesthetic that antagonizes the NMDA receptor. It has gained significant favor for use in the pediatric population thanks to its rapid onset, lack of respiratory depression, and efficacy at reducing pain within minutes. Of note, some institutions consider ketamine solely for sedation, which would be a relative barrier to administering it rapidly and readily for analgesic purposes, as sedation paperwork and monitoring would be necessitated in those practice environments. Lastly, though rare at analgesic or subdissociative dosages, the potential for emergence phenomenon should be considered and addressed with patients' parents/guardians so they can anticipate its possibility and therefore be less distressed.

Bringing together everything we have discussed and applying it to this case, a kind, gentle nurse quickly assesses his pain using the Wong-Baker faces scale, which he marks as hurts a " whole lot." He is allowed to sit in a position of comfort in triage on his mom's lap with his arm elevated, a splint is placed, and he is offered a dose of PO ibuprofen and/or acetaminophen. LMX cream is applied to his bilateral upper extremities. The right (unaffected) extremity will be the site of IV placement and the left upper extremity will be the site of a hematoma block if needed during closed reduction of the fracture. He is given IN fentanyl, and his pain is reassessed and is now at "hurts little bit." Since analgesia is sufficiently achieved at this point, x-rays can be obtained followed by IV placement for labs and additional analgesia as needed. Reduction of the displaced fractures can be achieved using ketamine and a hematoma block with 2% lidocaine. The patient can most likely be discharged for orthopedic follow up with PO ibuprofen 10 mg/kg every 6 hours for 5 days in conjunction with acetaminophen 15 mg/kg every 4 hours and possibly oxycodone as needed for breakthrough pain, though this is often not required.

KEY POINTS TO REMEMBER

- Pediatric patients do not necessarily express pain the same way adults do, so continuous evaluation and reevaluation of potential pain in these patients is prudent. Use of pediatric pain scores can help facilitate and standardize this.
- Be proactive and preemptive about treating moderate to severe pain. If IV placement or invasive procedures are anticipated, consider early use of topical anesthetic creams such as LMX or EMLA at least 30–60 minutes prior when possible.
- Do not shy from using opioid medications when indicated, but do consider coadministering nonopioids such as acetaminophen and NSAIDs whenever possible to help reduce the amount of opioids required.
- Codeine should be avoided in pediatric patients due to variable and unpredictable metabolism.
- Consider IN analgesics in place of or as a bridge to parenteral analgesics as they have a quick onset and are less invasive.
- Consider alternating or combining analgesic classes to avoid maxing out on dosage.

Further Reading

AboutKidsHealth. Tools for measuring pain. https://www.aboutkidshealth.ca/Article?c ontentid=2994&language=English. Accessed February 6, 2019.

Baker CM, Wong DL. Q.U.E.S.T.: a process of pain assessment in children. *Orthop Nurs.* 1987;6(1):11–21.

Blondell RD, Azadfard M, Wisniewski AM. Pharmacologic therapy for acute pain. *Am Fam Physician.* 2013;87(11):766–72.

Children's Hospitals and Clinics of Minnesota. Pediatric acute pain management. Department of Medicine, Palliative Care, and Integrative Medicine. https://umanitoba.ca/faculties/health_sciences/medicine/units/pediatrics/media/2015_Pain_reference_printable_flyer.pdf. Accessed February 7, 2019.

Cohen LL, Lemanek K, Blount RL, et al. Evidence-based assessment of pediatric pain. *J Pediatr Psychol.* 2008;33(9):939–55.

Fox SM. Intranasal analgesia. *Pediatric EM Morsels.* https://pedemmorsels.com/intranasal-analgesia/. Accessed February 7, 2019.

Fox SM. Ketamine for analgesia. *Pediatric EM Morsels.* https://pedemmorsels.com/ketamine-analgesia/. Accessed February 7, 2019.

University of Wisconsin Health. Health facts for you: using pediatric pain scales. https://www.uwhealth.org/healthfacts/pain/7590.pdf. Accessed February 6, 2019.

Walker G, Arnold R. Palliative Care Network of Wisconsin. Fast facts and concepts #117: pediatric pain assessment scales. https://www.mypcnow.org/blank-kx3g3. Accessed February 6, 2019.

Williams J, Wharton R, Peev P, Horwitz M. Acute flexor tendon injury following midshaft radius and ulna fractures in a paediatric patient. 2018. Available at https://www.sciencedirect.com/science/article/pii/S2352644018300074. Accessed February 6, 2019.

20 The Neverending Ouch

Julianne Hughes and Isabel A. Barata

A 6-year-old male with a history of sickle cell disease presents to the emergency department with bilateral leg pain that has worsened over the last 4 days. The pain began in his lower extremities and has now spread to his knees and thighs. His parents were treating him with acetaminophen every 4 hours and ibuprofen every 6 hours without improvement in his pain; his prescription for oxycodone ran out. He is unable to ambulate and has pain at rest (pain score is 9/10). He has a history of frequent vaso-occlusive crises and poor adherence with his medications; forgetting to take his hydroxyurea weekly. He denies fever, respiratory symptoms, and abdominal pain. He has a heart rate of 98 bpm, a temperature of 37.1°C, blood pressure of 100/65, a respiratory rate of 22 breaths per minute, and an oxygen saturation of 99% on room air. On exam, his lower extremities are tender with limited range of motion secondary to pain (no warmth, edema or erythema of any joints). The rest of his exam is normal.

What do you do now?

CHRONIC PAIN

Diagnosis

This patient is having a vaso-occlusive crisis secondary to suboptimal management of his sickle cell disease. Vaso-occlusive crises are a result of occlusion of blood vessels by sickled red blood cells, resulting in ischemic tissue injury and episodes of extreme pain. Vaso-occlusive crises account for 79% to 91% of emergency department visits for patients with sickle cell disease. Chronic, but episodic, pain may occur in other chronic illnesses such as malignancy, inflammatory bowel disease, and juvenile idiopathic arthritis. Pain can also define the disorder itself, as in patients with migraines, functional abdominal pain, or complex regional pain syndrome. These patients are more likely to have persistent, or ongoing pain.

Chronic pain is defined as pain that is either persistent (ongoing) or recurrent (episodic) and is thought to be multifactorial, involving biological, psychological and sociocultural factors. Generally, pain is considered chronic when the pain itself or recurrent episodes of pain persist longer than 3 to 6 months. A pain-related presenting complaint accounts for up to 78% of pediatric emergency department visits, with an estimated 10% to 15% of those cases related to chronic pain disorders.

When considering the management of pain in a child with a chronic pain disorder, such as this child, assessment of pain is critical. In children without chronic pain disorders, it may be prudent to assess acute episodes of pain with physiologic changes such as a change in vital signs (tachycardia, tachypnea, hypertension, oxygen desaturation), increased muscle tone, diaphoresis, flushing, and/or pallor. Behavioral changes can also be assessed in such patients, including a change in facial expression, grimacing, writhing, sleep disturbances, or change in appetite. However, it is important to recognize that these clinical features of acute pain may not be present in patients with underlying chronic pain disorders. On initial assessment, a child's pain should be assessed and documented using validated tools based on the child's age, development, and ability to communicate. For younger children, a pictorial-based pain scale is most effective, such as the Wong-Baker FACES Pain Rating Scale or the OUCHER Pain Scale. Children greater than 8 years old can generally comply with the verbal numerical scales used in adults.

Once pain is initially assessed, treatment can be initiated based on the severity, nature, and presumed etiology of the pain. Management of acute or chronic pain episodes should follow evidence-based recommendations, which include both pharmacological and nonpharmacological principles. Unfortunately, most principles of chronic pain management are extrapolated from trials in adults, and there is very little evidence regarding the efficacy of such management in children. Special care should be taken in treating patients with chronic pain disorders who are experiencing acute pain flares or episodes secondary to their illness, as the patient may have developed tolerance to certain classes of drugs.

Pharmacologic analgesic therapy is warranted for all children with pain, assuming nonpharmacological approaches are insufficient or unlikely to achieve pain relief alone. Care should be taken when treating pain in children with chronic pain disorders, as they notoriously receive suboptimal analgesic dosing and are less likely to receive multimodal pain management than adults. This is of particular importance in patients with chronic pain disorders. These patients may have developed opioid tolerance secondary to recurrent or persistent pain, as this child has. In these cases, consider initiating pain management at higher doses than you would for a previously healthy patient. Checking the medical record for previous doses of medication that have been effective can also be helpful. Initiation of intravenous medication should be considered sooner than is typical, so that higher doses can be more rapidly titrated.

The first consideration of adequate pain management is the route of administration. In the emergency department, pediatric patients typically receive pain medication intranasally, orally, intramuscularly, or intravenously. When deciding on a route of administration, providers should consider the speed of onset, bioavailability, and the clinical scenario. Intranasal medications have a quicker onset and a higher bioavailability, but are of limited use in patients with nasal trauma or obstruction. Oral medications are usually the least traumatic, but have a slower onset and may be of limited use if the patient is vomiting or if fasting is indicated. Intravenously administered medications are best for treating severe pain, but come with challenges of achieving access. In this child with recurrent pain, topical agents may be placed at potential intravenous sites in triage, allowing for more painless intravenous access, which would be clearly the best route for administration in this child.

When deciding on what medication to use for treating pain, consider the severity of the pain (Table 20.1). For mild pain (a pain score of 1 to 3), begin with oral medications such as acetaminophen or nonsteroidal anti-inflammatory drugs (NSAIDs) like ibuprofen or naproxen. Both classes of drugs have been shown to provide adequate pain control, and when coadministered they can provide superior pain control as compared to either agent alone. Ibuprofen and naproxen are similar in their efficacy and mechanism of action, but naproxen may be used in cases where a longer-acting formula is desired. Often in children with chronic pain disorders, longer-acting formulas are preferred because of the chronic and recurrent nature of their pain (though keep mind naproxen is limited to patients over 2 years old). Special attention should be given to the risk of gastrointestinal bleeding with NSAID use, particularly when using longer-acting formulas, as the risk of gastrointestinal bleeding is higher. In children, aspirin is often avoided due to the risk of Reye's syndrome. However, when

TABLE 20.1. **Pain Management Based on Severity**

Pain Severity	Pain Score	Treatment Options
Mild	1–3	Acetaminophen (oral) Ibuprofen Naproxen
Moderate	4–6	Acetaminophen (intravenous) Fentanyl (intranasal) Hydrocodone Hydromorphone Ketorolac Oxycodone
Severe	7–10	Fentanyl (intravenous) Hydromorphone (intravenous) Morphine (intravenous)

treating patients with chronic pain disorders, particularly rheumatologic disorders, aspirin may be an appropriate agent. This child has already been receiving the maximum doses for these medications and so a more potent agent is needed.

Moderate pain (pain score 4–6) requires escalation of pain management. It is appropriate for providers to begin with pain control agents that are typically used for mild pain (acetaminophen, NSAIDs), but it is important to optimize pain control with dual modalities of pain management. Second-line treatment involves oral opioids, such as hydrocodone, oxycodone, or hydromorphone. Be sure to consider that some of these medications are already dual modality medications. For example, Vicodin and Percocet contain combinations of acetaminophen and hydrocodone and oxycodone respectively. It is prudent to recognize the exact contents of your chosen pain medication to prevent an excessive dose of acetaminophen.

Other second-line treatments include intranasal medications such as fentanyl or diamorphine. These medications are limited to pediatric patients over 6 months old. Intravenous forms of mild pain management agents, such as acetaminophen or ketorolac, may also be used to achieve pain control in patients with moderate pain.

For severe pain (pain score 7–10), such as the child in this scenario, intravenous access should be obtained without delay. If there is a delay in obtaining access, intranasal medications can be given as temporary pain relief. Also consider the application of topical agents to potential intravenous access sites in triage to decrease the pain associated with obtaining access. Intravenous opioids should be used with severe pain, such as morphine, fentanyl, or hydromorphone. Special care should be taken when treating severe pain with intravenous opioids, including cardiac and respiratory status monitoring, because of the rare, but dangerous side effect of respiratory depression. Though unlikely, if respiratory depression becomes severe, resuscitation and naloxone therapy should be initiated.

Nonpharmacologic pain management should be integrated with pharmacologic pain management to ensure optimal pain control. Physical, psychological, and behavioral modifications can be used adjunctively to improve treatment of chronic pain in the emergency department. These interventions, when integrated in an age-appropriate manner, can assist in improving the fears and stressors surrounding the patient's pain.

Two strategies for the nonpharmacologic treatment of pain are recommended: physical comfort measures and distracting measures. For neonates and younger patients, there is evidence that physical comfort measures decrease distress during pain episodes and provide a positive physiologic response (decreased pain scores, decreased crying). Some options for patients in this age group include oral stimulation, swaddling, or being touched. Children outside of infancy often benefit from distracting measures or activities. These vary based on age but can include music, interactive games, books, or deep breathing exercises. For older children, the application of cold or hot packs for minor injuries may be effective. For patients with chronic pain who are cognitively impaired, environmental considerations should take particular precedence. Working with parents to discuss comfort strategies that have previously been successful, or strategies to avoid, is important. This child enjoys playing games on his mother's phone, and the nurse is able to locate a charging cord to allow the child to play games while pharmacologic therapy is initiated.

When attempting pain management in the emergency department, consider assistance from an integrative pain team (when available). These teams may consist of anesthesiologists, palliative care specialists, or physiatrists. They are equipped to assist in providing options for multimodal pain management, particular in patients with chronic pain disorders. They are also helpful when a patient requires additional pain services, such as physical or occupational therapy. Other members of these teams may include child life specialists, art therapists, music therapists, massage therapists, and/or those trained in spiritual or emotional support.

A key component of effective pain management lies with periodic reassessment of pain. Your initial assessment should guide your treatment of pain in the emergency department, but it is important to establish the effectiveness of your chosen treatment. Using the "score, treat, score" method for patients allows you to adjust your management plan according to its effectiveness and the clinical scenario. When reassessing pain, consider the patient's underlying diagnosis and implement condition-specific management plans. This patient receives an intravenous dose of fentanyl which on reassessment has reduced his pain score to 5 out of 10. For patients with chronic pain disorders, consider involving specialty services that may be of assistance with their long-term, discharge plan. Pain specialists or anesthesiologists may provide alternative therapies to prevent hospital admission or return to the emergency department.

Discharge criteria for patients with a chronic pain disorder can be challenging to determine. For patients that are chronic pain sufferers, it is important to have an understanding of their baseline status. Goals should center around improving functionality and quality of life, not necessarily using pain intensity as a marker, but instead using functional indicators of improvement. Patients with cognitive impairment may have patterns of episodic pain that are typical for them. Referrals and discharge planning is key to help prevent return emergency department visits. These patients may require services such as physical, occupational, or psychological therapies. This child receives a second dose of fentanyl and is admitted to the hospital for pain control and patient education.

Better education about home pain management is critical in improving pain outcomes for children with chronic pain disorders, such as this child. While it appears that the parents and patient were educated about stepwise treatment and the nature of his episodic pain episodes associated with his chronic pain disorder, they did not seem to understand the value of the hydroxyurea. He was appropriately taking ibuprofen at the first signs of pain, and the parents knew to escalate to his second-line treatment of oxycodone for refractory pain. Ideally in this scenario, they would have ensured through their outpatient hematology visits that he had an adequate supply of his medications for his home medical management. Another consideration was this patient's difficulty with medical adherence. He had not been taking his hydroxyurea as instructed, which he was prescribed to help prevent his frequent pain crises. In this case, education and support of pain management at discharge is essential to prevent further pain episodes. Parents should be thoroughly educated regarding the appropriate frequency and dose of both prophylactic and breakthrough pain medication. Ultimately, outpatient management is a key component for managing chronic pain, so care should be taken in ensuring reliable follow-up.

· Clinical features of acute pain may not be present in patients with chronic pain disorders.

· Obtain initial pain scores and use these to help guide your pain management.

· Patients with chronic pain may require higher doses, or different routes of administration than patients without chronic pain disorders.

· Nonpharmacologic pain management should be used adjunctively with pharmacologic pain management.

· A key component of effective pain management lies with periodic reassessment of pain.

· Ultimately, education and outpatient management are key, so care should be taken in ensuring reliable follow-up.

Further Reading

American Pain Society. Assessment and management of children with chronic pain. A position statement from the American Pain Society. 2012. Available at: http://americanpainsociety.org/uploads/get-involved/pediatric-chronic-pain-statement.pdf.

Feldman K, Berall A, Karuza J, Senderovich H, Perri G-A, Grossman D. Knowledge translation: an interprofessional approach to integrating a pain consult team within an acute care unit. *J Interprofess Care*. 2016;30(6):816–8. doi:10.1080/13561820.2016.1195342.

Friedrichsdorf S, Giordano J, Dakoji KD, Warmuth A, Daughtry C, Schulz C. Chronic pain in children and adolescents: diagnosis and treatment of primary pain disorders in head, abdomen, muscles and joints. *Children*. 2016;3(4):42. doi:10.3390/children3040042.

Krauss BS, Calligaris L, Green SM, Barbi E. Current concepts in management of pain in children in the emergency department. *Lancet*. 2016;387(10013):83–92. doi:10.1016/s0140-6736(14)61686-x.

Motov SM, Nelson LS. Advanced concepts and controversies in emergency department pain management. *Anesthesiol Clin*. 2016;34(2):271–85. doi:10.1016/j.anclin.2016.01.006.

Poulin PA, Nelli J, Tremblay S, et al. Chronic pain in the emergency department: a pilot mixed-methods cross-sectional study examining patient characteristics and reasons for presentations. *Pain Res Manage*. 2016;2016:1–10. doi:10.1155/2016/3092391.

21 Am I Safe?

Elizabeth A. Berdan and
Elizabeth A. Woods

"Sarah" is a 15-year-old girl who presents to your emergency department (ED) after being found disoriented at a city bus stop by a passerby. She was brought to the ED by law enforcement. On your initial exam she is disoriented, and she appears to be under the influence of a mind-altering substance(s). She is frightened, and her hair and clothing are disheveled. It is difficult to get an accurate history from Sarah, as her speech is not coherent and her thought process is guarded, defensive, and tangential. The police report to you that Sarah was found in their database as a runaway, and there is a warrant for her arrest for "something minor."

What do you do now?

PATIENT INTERVIEW AND OUTCOME

When you question Sarah further, she confirmed she ran away 3 weeks ago because she was suspended from school for marijuana use. She has been staying with a "friend". Sarah disclosed that she escaped today and explained the scratches and bruising on her arms were obtained as a result of trying to escape. Between investigator information and a brief disclosure from the patient, it became clear that Sarah, following her voluntary departure from home, had been sex trafficked. All interviewing ceased and the child abuse consultant at the Children's Advocacy Center (CAC) was notified, who discouraged any further interviewing of the patient so a forensic interview could be scheduled. Based on the patient's disorientation, inability to consent to a sexual assault exam, and a positive drug screen (+methamphetamines and cannabinoids), further evaluation was delayed until the following day. After an overnight stay in the ED, arrangements were made for the patient to be seen at the CAC. At the CAC she received a forensic interview and physical exam, including a colposcopic exam, and sexual assault exam with collection of evidence. A local patient advocacy group for victims of sex trafficking was emergently notified and an advocate was assigned to the patient to provide ongoing compassionate care with other community entities including Department of Children, Youth & Families, law enforcement, and the prosecuting attorney's office. The advocacy group provided their services in the hospital during Sarah's hospitalization and remained involved with the patient post-hospitalization.

Sarah ultimately reported approximately 20–30 sexual encounters over several weeks. At the time of her initial ED presentation Sarah did not identify herself as a victim and insisted that she was in charge of all the incidents that occurred in the preceding weeks. She wanted to return to her traffickers. She requested information from law enforcement about her perpetrators and voiced concern regarding their arrests. Sarah reported a difficult home life and implied it was worse than what she experienced by the traffickers. She begged her health care professionals (HCPs) and law enforcement not to send her back home. Eventually Sarah returned home and has since spoken publicly against her traffickers and the horrors of sex trafficking. Ultimately 4 individuals were arrested and charged with kidnapping, rape of a child, providing drugs to a minor, promoting sex abuse of a minor, and sex trafficking.

WARNING

Most victims of sex trafficking will not announce their victimization to you. You have to look carefully. You have to ask the difficult, probing questions. You may not even obtain a disclosure of trafficking victimization. Outcomes are often not as successful as in the case described. Sex trafficking of children is an uncomfortable topic. The treatment of trauma induced by the heinous violations sustained by this patient population requires a multidisciplinary team approach. The first step, the most important step, is recognition of what is behind the chief complaint.

BACKGROUND

While there is a growing body of research that describes the pervasive public health issue of human trafficking (HT), many HCPs do not recognize signs of HT in their patients; thereby missing an opportunity for intervention.[1,2] This is not surprising given that despite federal law, which defines the victims of HT as just that—victims and NOT offenders, many victims of HT are incarcerated for crimes related to their exploitation. The United Nations defines acts of trafficking in persons as the "recruitment, transportation, transfer, harboring or receipt of persons, by means of the threat or use of force or other forms of coercion, of abduction, of fraud, of deception, of the abuse of power or of a position of vulnerability or of the giving or receiving of payments or benefits to achieve the consent of a person having control over another person for the purpose of exploitation." If the victim is under the age of 18 the elements of "force, fraud, coercion, deception, or other means of abuse power" need not be required to meet the definition of child sex trafficking. In other words, engaging a minor in any form of sex act in return for something of value is a serious violation of human rights. The interaction of HCPs with trafficking victims offers an opportunity for intervention; however, HCPs are missing the opportunity for motivational interviewing, harm reduction, and preventive measures. These missed opportunities are the result of a knowledge deficit in the recognition of, and lack of experience with providing trauma-informed care to, patients who are victims of trafficking.

The identification of trafficking victims is complicated by layers of variables. Fearful of incarceration, and often treated as criminals, victims/survivors of trafficking may not actively seek supportive services. Furthermore, a victim of trafficking is not likely to self-identify as a victim owing to the deceptive and coercive nature of the psychological trauma inflicted by the trafficker as the trafficker "grooms" the victim to believe they are friends of, girlfriends of, and/or loved by the trafficker. This grooming results in a powerful trauma-bond between the trafficker and their victim, leading to fierce loyalty. Traffickers use threats, punishments, and lies to frighten victims into silence. Even if the exploited individual recognizes their victimization, their fear of, or loyalty to, their trafficker may be a barrier to disclosure. Feelings of shame, humiliation, and fear of harsh judgment from HCPs may cause reluctance to disclose their circumstances, with many insisting that they behaved voluntarily.[1,3]

The urgent care or ED (56%) setting is the prevailing venue for the intersection between healthcare and trafficking.[2,4] Restricting access to medical care is a mechanism of control used by the trafficker. Thus, minor infections or illnesses are often left untreated until they become urgent or emergent. Trafficking victims also seek care at a surprising rate in primary care (44%), subspecialty, and dental (27%) clinics.[2,4] Reasons care is sought may be directly related to their trafficking experience such as an acute traumatic injury, mental health crisis, severe infection, or drug overdose.[4] Furthermore, we know trafficked individuals also seek care for conditions unrelated to their current trafficking situation such as appendicitis, viral illnesses, heart concerns, and complications with preexisting conditions.[4] While there are risk factors associated with sex trafficking victimization (see Table 21.1),[3] these are not necessarily causal. Some patients have no risk factors other than their youth, which simply highlights an adolescent's proclivity for risk-taking and impulsivity as a result of their neurodevelopmental stage. This underscores the unique vulnerability of children and adolescents.

The mental and physical health consequences as a result of the severity of, nature of, and repetition of trauma have devastating effects. The adverse health effects of sexually exploited children include violent acute traumatic injuries, sexually transmitted infections (STIs), pregnancy, untreated chronic illness, substance abuse, complex post-traumatic stress disorder, major depression, suicidality, anxiety, and co-occurring behavioral problems of self-harm and cutting.[3,5,6]

PATIENT AND HEALTHCARE PROFESSIONAL INTERACTION

Establish a Trusting Relationship

A disclosure of being trafficked is not the goal, rather the goal is to identify risk factors (Table 21.2) and limit the potential harm. To ensure that trust is not broken, inform your patient of your requirement by law to notify authorities if they report information that indicates they are being harmed or their life is at risk.[7] Be cautious in presuming that law enforcement and/or the Department of Children, Youth & Families are equipped to provide safety and resources. Engage a local patient advocacy group for victims of sex trafficking so the child will have a trained advocate and access to necessary resources. Many community entities are not yet trained, nor do they have adequate resources for sex trafficking victims/survivors.

Listen to the patient and see them as an individual; support them in the choices they make, and help them to see that choices do in fact exist. All patients should be treated as victims/survivors and not criminals. The services they receive should be "victim"-centered. Patients must be treated with respect, be asked to share their views, and be given choices as much as possible. Family members, caregivers, and friends should be included when possible in service and planning efforts.

Interview, Exam, and Documentation

You must *interview the patient alone* and inform the patient of your mandatory reporting obligations. Once red flags for possible sex trafficking victimization have been identified you may use probing questions such as, "Do you feel up to telling me what happened?"[8] Once a pediatric patient is identified as having a current or past history of being trafficked it is critical to stop further interviewing and refer to a facility capable of performing a child forensic interview, which reduces the number of interviews conducted and minimizes trauma.

TABLE 21.1.   **Risk Factors Associated with Child Sex Trafficking Victimization**

Risk Factors[3]

History of sexual abuse
History of foster care
LGBTQ youth
Runaway youth
Throwaway youth (forced to leave home or not allowed to return home)
Homeless youth
Intellectually disabled
History of dating violence
History of rape and sexual assault
History of incarceration, juvenile justice, or child protective service
Some patients have no risk factors other than their youth

Note: LGBTQ = Lesbian, gay, bisexual, transgender, queer/questioning.

Sexual Assault Exams

Exams by a trained provider and/or Sexual Assault Nurse Examiner (SANE)[9] should be provided to:

1. any patient who has experienced sexual assault in the preceding 120 hours. These patients require an acute exam and forensic evidence collection.
2. any patient experiencing symptoms.
3. any patient who has concerns about their body (this does not require an acute exam).

Consent is required. Any of the above patients may decline a sexual assault exam, and their decision must be respected. We do not want to retraumatize an already traumatized individual. An individual under the influence of drugs or alcohol (as in the patient described) or mentally unstable is incapable of consent. A sexual assault exam must be delayed until consent can be attained.

Questions asked during the medical exam of a child should remain limited strictly to medical concerns and the patient's safety. Spontaneous disclosures by a child to a HCP should be documented with quotes. Consider a response of "I am so glad you told me, and I am going to help you get the help you need. I am going to help get all the right people on

TABLE 21.2. **Red Flags for Sex Trafficking**

History	Exam
Untreated chronic conditions	Signs of drug abuse
Multiple pregnancies/terminations	Sexually explicit tattoos, gang symbols, barcodes
Minor with a companion who will not leave	Somatic manifestations of stress
Multiple STIs	Fearful, anxious, and/or depressed affect
Minor present without a legal guardian	Inappropriately dressed for weather
Lack of knowledge of location	Have items seemingly too expensive for socioeconomic class
Inconsistent story	Vaginal and/or rectal lacerations
Unclear housing situation	May have 2 cell phones, or hold cell phone in lab for entire visit
Truancy from school	
Multiple sexual partners	

Note: This is not an exhaustive list of possible indicators, which should be taken in context, and presence of these indicators is not to be considered "proof" that sex trafficking is occurring.

your team who know how to best care for you. I will take care of your medical needs and ensure we get the best help we can."

The Role of a Children's Advocacy Center
Collaboration with your local or regional CAC in cases involving the commercial sexual exploitation of children may be critical to the successful navigation of safety concerns, appropriate treatment, interviewing, investigation, and placement of a child.

Local Patent Advocacy
Partnering with local advocacy organizations for victims of sex trafficking may be an important aspect of connecting patients to the resources and community needed for recovery. The goal of patient advocacy models is to provide a nonjudgmental, confidential advocacy role to support the

individual with compassion and provide access to critical community resources (job training/placement, education, safe houses, etc.).

Discharge Planning

Not all suspicious interactions will result in a disclosure of trafficking victimization. Discharge and follow-up is the responsibility of the HCP. Patient safety is the paramount concern.

- Verbally provide the patient with the number to the National Trafficking Hotline (1-888-373-7888) and ask them to repeat the number back to you. It is easy to remember the number "888–3737–888." They can also text "help" to BeFree.
- Obtain an accurate contact number for the patient, AND for two additional people who are in contact with the patient.
- Perhaps provide the patient a written appointment to "return to the doctor for an X-ray."

One option is to have several outpatient providers trained in the evaluation and support of victims. Discharges from the ED or inpatient services can be directed to these providers who offer long-term plans and physician–patient relationship building. Without a team of outpatient providers trained in the evaluation and support of victims an ED HCP is left with an approach of "if you need help come to the ED and if I'm here I will help you or one of my colleagues will. We will always be on your side." We must support the change in our community and consider that when our system does not support safe and effective patient care, it is our responsibility to fill that role.

CONCLUSION

Many survivors report being harshly judged and treated when they are seen in the ED.[4] Others report that they presented for care and no one asked the uncomfortable questions. HCPs may make a substantial impact if we are prepared to identify sex trafficking of minors and treat the victims with dignity and compassion, and we have resources to offer. We must avoid thinking that we can "rescue" these individuals.

In order to recognize and prevent the sexual exploitation of children a culture change is needed with prioritization of better funded services for the care of exploited children. Education of providers in EDs and all health-care settings is a priority. Posting of educational tools, emergency hotline numbers in our hospitals and clinics, and guidelines could be lifesaving. Establishing guidelines for the screening and evaluation of these patients may impact safe outcomes for victims/survivors of human trafficking. Engage your local child abuse consultants, CAC, Commercial Sexual Exploitation of Children (CSEC) committees, and local community resources to stop the sexual exploitation of children and adults.

KEY POINTS TO REMEMBER

- Treat the patient respectfully, without judgment, and with compassion.
- Build trust with the patient by identifying your mandatory reporting obligations BEFORE you ask questions.
- Patient safety as your largest concern.
- Once a patient is suspected of being trafficked, engage your local CAC, and determine a safety plan.
- Seek community resources and establish a follow-up plan.
- Educate your community.
- Develop a hospital guideline for the screening, treatment, and evaluation of these patients.
- Collaborate with local institutions, community entities, and resources.

List of Educational Resources
American Medical Association: AMA on HT
American Medical Women's Association—Physicians Against the Trafficking
    of Humans
Dignity Health: Human Trafficking Response
HEAL Trafficking: Education and Training Committee
Health & Human Services: SOAR

Further Reading

1. Lederer LJ, Wetzel CA, Health T. The health consequences of sex trafficking and their implications for identifying victims in healthcare facilities. *Ann Health Law*. 2014;23:61.

2. Chisolm-Straker M, Baldwin S, Gaïgbé-Togbé B, Ndukwe N, Johnson PN, Richardson LD. Health care and human trafficking: we are seeing the unseen. *J Health Care Poor Underserved*. 2016;27(3):1220–33. doi:10.1353/hpu.2016.0131.

3. Greenbaum J, Crawford-Jakubiak JE. Child sex trafficking and commercial sexual exploitation: health care needs of victims. *Pediatrics*. 2015;135(3):566–74. doi:10.1542/peds.2014-4138.

4. Polaris Project Report. *On-Ramps, Intersections, and Exit Routes: A Roadmap for Systems and Industries to Prevent and Disrupt Human Trafficking*. 2018:1–176. https://polarisproject.org/wp-content/uploads/2018/08/A-Roadmap-for-Systems-and-Industries-to-Prevent-and-Disrupt-Human-Trafficking.pdf

5. Simkhada P, van Teijlingen E, Sharma A, Bissell P, Poobalan A, Wasti SP. Health consequences of sex trafficking: a systematic review. *J Manmohan Mem Instit Health Sci* 2018;4(1). doi:10.3126/jmmihs.v4i1.21150.

6. Flaherty E, Legano L, Idzerda S. Ongoing pediatric health care for the child who has been maltreated. *Pediatrics*. 2019;143(4):e20190284. doi:10.1542/peds.2019-0284.

7. Barnert E, Iqbal Z, Bruce J, Anoshiravani A, Kolhatkar G, Greenbaum J. Commercial sexual exploitation and sex trafficking of children and adolescents: a narrative review. *Academic Pediatrics*. 2017;17(8):825–9. doi:10.1016/j.acap.2017.07.009.

8. Lyman M, Borham K, Berdan E, Geynisman J, Gordon M, DiPaolo C, Martinez K, Titchen K. LIFT: Learn, Identify, Fight Trafficking Course. *American Medical Womens Association -Physicians Against the Trafficking of Humans (AMWA-PATH)*. 2019. https://www.amwa-doc.org/our-work/initiatives/human-trafficking/

9. Crawford-Jakubiak JE, Alderman EM, Leventhal JM. Care of the adolescent after an acute sexual assault. *Pediatrics*. 2017;139(3). doi:10.1542/peds.2016-4243

Index

Tables and figures are indicated by *t* and *f* following the page number